# HormoneSynergy

*Optimal aging and hormone balance*

# HormoneSynergy

*Optimal aging and hormone balance*

Kathryn Retzler, ND

*To Leanna,*
*You are a spunky,*
*vibrant woman!*
*With gratitude,*
*Kathryn*

HormoneSynergy®

Paperback ISBN 978-0-557-37056-6

Hardcover ISBN 978-0-557-37057-3

# HormoneSynergy®

*Optimal aging and hormone balance*

## Author's Note

*To my greatest cheerleaders (my mother, Debbie, and my husband, Daniel) and to all the generous people who trust me with their health and enable me to perform my calling*

# Acknowledgments

I am deeply grateful to many people who've taught, inspired, and supported me on my journey to becoming a physician, and in my quest to share the knowledge I've acquired with anyone who will listen. My mentor, Dr. Rebecca Glaser, deserves special mention for allowing me open access to her immense treasure of data on bioidentical hormones and breast cancer, and for her tireless commitment to research regarding the benefits of testosterone for women (you are my hero!) Dr. Alison McAllister, with her brilliant brain and comprehension of biochemistry and hormones, has been a charitable teacher and resource. For her inspiration, kind words, and unconditional soothing of my soul, Dr. Sherry LaBeck deserves my gratitude. Dr. Bruce Dickson, thank you for your faith in me when I was your resident. For sharing his wealth of information about hormones and for allowing me to play a short part in his vision, I am thankful to Dr. David Zava. Dr. Elizabeth Sutherland, I wouldn't be the same, personally or professionally, without your enormous influence in my life.

Of course, writing a book while maintaining a busy practice requires sacrifice, diligence, and a continual source of unconditional support; that support is my husband, Daniel. To my mother, Debbie, and step-father, Mike, who've always found a way to assist in my education and work, thank you for believing in me. As a struggling medical student, Jean, Jay, William, and Sarah provided me shelter and unconditional love. I appreciate all the help I've received from my father, Bob, and my step-mom, Betsy. And to my in-laws, Carol and Jay, I'm humbled by your love and admiration.

# Contents

# Introduction

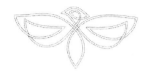

In old school, conventional medicine, you were a "patient "—a word based on the Latin *patiens*, "one who endures or suffers calmly or without complaint"—the same root that gives us the word "passive."

You are not passive any longer.

As I write this, we are in the midst of a paradigm shift in medicine. Doctors are increasingly embracing their role as teachers, and all of us as "patients" are rejecting passivity and embracing our role as captains of our fate and masters of our lives—as empowered partners in the search for vibrant health.

By seeking out information—including the information found in this book—you are taking responsibility for your own health. And by accepting the happy burden of knowledge, of understanding how your body works, you gain the fundamental ability to create a healthy life.

When you translate the knowledge you acquire from this book into action, you will not only slow your rate of aging and reduce your risk for chronic disease, you will also save a lot of money. Consider the current average cost of long-term care according to the American Association of Retired People: $206 per day for a private room in a nursing home or $98 per day for an assisted living unit. That's $35,000 to $75,000 per year for long-term care. Can you afford this? Can your family?

Be forewarned: by embracing the optimal aging strategies found in this book, you will diminish the enormous profits of the pharmaceutical industry. In 2007, the American pharmaceutical industry sold $300 billion dollars worth of drugs, and made more than $100 billion in profits. The average Medicare patient takes four drugs every day. Only 11 percent of Medicare patients use no drugs—while 25% of Medicare patients take six or more medications. How many medications are you on, and how many are you willing to tolerate?

Aging isn't optional, but you <u>can</u> choose to experience optimal aging. At times, you may travel through the land of symptoms and disease; you may even need medications to manage health problems. But you know that, beyond the place marked by the mere absence of symptoms or disease, is another realm of truly vibrant health.

Although many cosmetic companies claim that anti-aging is as simple as using a special cream or skin treatment, this approach is like painting over rust—eventually the rust breaks through. To experience vibrant health, you must start at the cellular level.

If you're committed to taking responsibility for your health, to start slowing or reversing the aging process at the cellular level, you'll need to be open to new information. This information must include an understanding of your own hormones—how hormones affect your health, and how you can achieve hormone balance. And if you're searching for truly vibrant health and optimal aging—more than the mere absence of symptoms or disease—this book will serve as your map and compass.

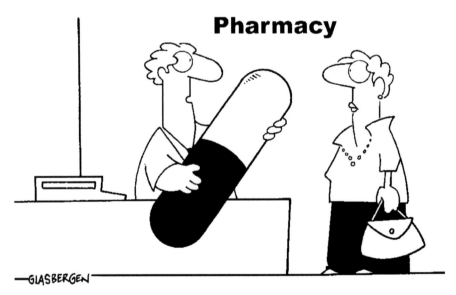

"Each capsule contains your medication,
plus a treatment for each of its side effects."

### *How this book is organized*

First, I'll discuss basic information about how aging happens and what hormones do. The first three chapters are followed by "Points to Remember" — these summarize concepts for you to take into following chapters to understand symptoms of imbalance and treatment options.

**Chapter 1** briefly describes *how aging happens.*

**Chapter 2** explains *what hormones are*, what they do, the concept of "Hormone Synergy," and "The 5 HormoneSynergy Principles".

**Chapter 3** introduces *the major hormones* – estrogen, progesterone, testosterone, DHEA, cortisol, thyroid hormone, and insulin, and the functions they perform in your body. (Women and men make all of the same hormones, just in different amounts, so this information applies to everyone.)

**Chapter 4** discusses the *symptoms* that occur when hormones fall out of balance.

**Chapter 5** describes *testing* to determine a blueprint of your *hormone levels*. Although symptoms often guide which hormones need balancing, testing can confirm suspicions as well as provide key information for dosages and treatment. Other optimal aging tests — including *genetic susceptibility, telomere length, free radical levels, and antioxidant status* – will be reviewed.

**Chapter 6** outlines the *four main causes* of hormone imbalance — toxicity, poor diet and lifestyle habits, stress, and aging. This chapter contains *The 8 Steps to Achieving HormoneSynergy*, giving you specific tools and natural treatments that form the foundation for optimal aging.

**Chapter 7** reviews *benefits, risks, and research about bioidentical hormone replacement* as well as modes of delivery.

**Chapter 8** provides more information on bioidentical hormones, *breast cancer, and prostate cancer.*

**Chapter 9** includes an *Optimal Aging Questionnaire* as well as *resources* for you to learn more about how you can achieve HormoneSynergy.

I hope you enjoy this journey through one of the most exciting systems of your body, your endocrine, or hormone, system. This system has tremendous influence over who you are, how you feel, and whether you age gracefully—with a healthy brain, abundant energy, and vibrant health. Once you've read this book, you will be empowered to create the healthy life you desire, and deserve.

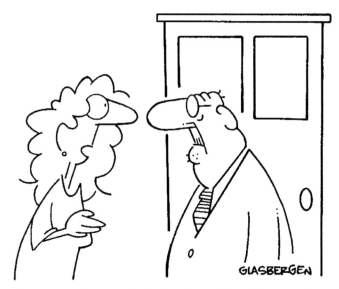

**"Honey, when you left for the office this morning, you were a happy, enthusiastic, vibrant 25 year old! Do you want to talk about it?"**

# Chapter 1: How Aging Happens

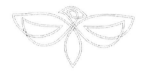

Many people feel like aging seems to happen overnight, that it's a process beyond their control. Tom and Linda held these beliefs when they first came to see me. Tom, a 56-year old engineer, explained his symptoms this way:

> *I'm not sure when I started to go downhill, but it's as if I woke up one day and realized I was getting old. My joints are stiff and creaky when I wake up, and I'm really tired by the time I get home. I used to be so sharp at work — I could figure out complex problems without much effort and my memory was quick. Now I have to struggle just to keep on task, and my mind is dull. My wife thinks I'm depressed, but I'm not sad — I just don't have the motivation or drive I used to. I've also put on weight. I don't really feel like working out or pushing myself to go to the gym — honestly, I'd rather just watch TV. I guess it's just downhill from here, part of getting old.*

Tom really believed his declining health and performance were inevitable, even at the youthful age of 56! Another patient, Linda, a 53-year-old emergency room nurse, held a similar belief:

> *When I first started going through menopause, I realized my youth was over. Before hot flashes, my sex drive was gone and I noticed my skin started sagging and the wrinkles multiplied. Sometimes when I'm at work, I forget what I'm doing, or I go to say something and the words evaporate. I've started relying on caffeine, chocolate, and sugar — whatever it takes to get through the day. By the time I get home, I'm so exhausted and crabby. I snap at my kids or husband for the smallest things. I don't even recognize myself anymore. I suppose I should accept all these problems as normal since I'm just getting older . . .*

I encourage you to recognize that, although health decline, lack of energy, thinning skin, weight gain, low libido, trouble thinking, and loss of joy are common, they are not necessarily normal—you don't have to accept them as consequences of aging. No matter what your doctor implies—falling apart as you age is not inevitable! Understanding how aging happens at the cellular level will provide a foundation for you to build a younger, healthier mind and body.

Although there are several theories about why we age, three of the most solid include telomere shortening, free radical damage, and declining hormone production.

### *Telomere Shortening*

To understand what telomeres are and how they affect aging, it's helpful to review what you learned in biology about your cells. You may recall that there are 46 chromosomes in each cell of your body (22 pairs plus the sex chromosomes, XX or XY). A chromosome is a single, very long piece of DNA. It may surprise you to know that more than 99% of human DNA is the same; in fact, only 0.1% of our DNA makes us unique individuals.

Segments of DNA, called "genes" act as instructions for your cells' activities. There are approximately 20,000 to 25,000 genes in the human genome—the map of human genes. The genes you've inherited, your unique genome, is often compared to a very long instruction manual or "book of life." If your book of life were printed, it would contain more than one billion words, written in 5000 volumes, each 300 pages long! A copy of this book—all of your DNA and genes—fits into the pinpoint-sized nucleus of nearly every one of your body's trillions of cells.

You may believe that genes determine your destiny and whether or not you develop certain health problems. However, this isn't necessarily true. Although you cannot change your genes, you can change how your genes express themselves. This is an area of research called "epigenetics." Epigenetics consists of how genes express themselves, including the influences of diet, lifestyle, and toxin exposure. So, what you eat, do, think, and surround yourself with, influences who you become in terms of appearance and health. In fact, longevity is thought to be at least 66% lifestyle choices.[1]

Your genes replicate themselves an average of 50 to 70 times before dying. Recall that genes are segments of DNA that makes up chromosomes. Chromosomes are protected on each end by regions known as "telomeres." Molecular biologist and Nobel Prize winner Elizabeth Blackburn has likened telomeres to aglets—the plastic pieces on the end of shoelaces that prevent them from unraveling. With each replication of a cell, telomeres shorten—the shorter your telomeres, the greater your biological age.

Certain conditions, such as eating an inflammatory diet high in processed food, sugar, trans fats, and animal products, will shorten telomeres faster. Telomere shortening is sped up by chronic stress, and sped up even more with free radical damage. Eating a healthy diet, taking antioxidants and vitamin D, and maintaining a healthy weight can help to lengthen telomeres. In addition, sleeping well, exercising, managing stress, and using bioidentical hormones can delay telomere shortening and the aging process (more on these optimal aging strategies in chapter 6).

## Free Radicals

Free radicals are atoms or molecules with unpaired electrons. Free radicals form as a byproduct of normal metabolism and can increase with sun exposure, cigarette smoking, or contact with toxins. Free radicals are dangerous because they cause chain reactions that damage DNA, proteins, and cells. If you imagine the excessive skin wrinkling of a cigarette smoker, you'd be viewing the damage to collagen by free radicals.

Similar to the way oxygen free radicals turn iron into rust, free radicals in the body accelerate aging. Free radical damage speeds up the aging of your skin, and has been linked to many forms of cancer, strokes, and atherosclerosis. In addition, free radicals contribute to the brain damage seen in Parkinson's and Alzheimer's disease. You can limit free radical damage to your cells by using antioxidants, such as vitamins A, C, E, coenzyme Q10, and selenium, all of which quench free radicals. More on testing for free radical damage and treatment in later chapters. For now, understand that free radicals can shorten telomeres and accelerate aging.

## Hormone Decline

Besides telomere shortening and free radical damage, hormone decline contributes to aging. Hormones are responsible for repair of tissues and regulation of cellular metabolism and function. Most hormones decline with age, and aging accelerates when hormone levels decline.

Humans are a unique species when it comes to the fact that we live much of our lives outside our reproductive years. Most animals in the wild do not live beyond their ability to reproduce — many don't even live beyond puberty. Our increased life expectancy is relatively recent— only women and men in the past few generations have a life expectancy beyond 60 years. There is certainly much controversy about whether or not it's appropriate to restore hormones to youthful levels as people age (this will be discussed in the BHRT chapter). However, most people will agree that signs of aging increase dramatically after their reproductive years (around age 40 or 45).

Although your telomeres shorten, free radical damage increases, and hormones decline over time, you can slow or reverse these processes by following *The 8 Steps to Achieving Hormone Synergy* introduced in chapter 6. Before jumping ahead, it's helpful to review what hormones are, what they do, and why they matter.

## Points to remember:

- Telomere shortening, free radical damage, and declining hormone levels all contribute to aging.
- Although genes are inherited, how your genes express themselves greatly influences your health and longevity. Diet, lifestyle, and toxicity all affect how your genes express themselves.
- There is much you can do to slow telomere shortening, quench free radicals, and optimize hormone levels (hint: follow *The 8 Steps to Achieving Hormone Synergy*).

# Chapter 2: What Hormones Are and What They Do

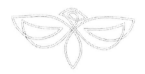

Hormones are chemicals made by glands that travel through the bloodstream and bind to receptors on or inside cells. For proper function, each hormone must fit the specific receptor it binds to, like a key in a lock. When the key and lock don't fit exactly, health problems can result. This is why your body's own hormones (or "bioidentical" hormones) are better than synthetic, foreign ones.

Hormones are often referred to as chemical messengers because they are the language that cells use to communicate. The word "hormone" comes from the Greek word "horman" which means "to set in motion"—an excellent description for the enormous job that hormones perform. Hormones play a direct or indirect role in nearly all your body's processes. This includes growth and development from childhood to adulthood, and the well-known role hormones play in reproduction. Hormones are also largely responsible for repairing your body's tissues—such as skin, muscle, and bone—which is why hormone decline can lead to sagging skin, decreased muscle mass and strength, and bone loss.

Hormones control the function of your immune system; hormone imbalance can contribute to the formation of allergies or autoimmune problems, as well as an increased risk for infections and developing cancer. Certain hormones determine blood sugar regulation and the ability to maintain healthy blood sugar levels decreases with aging. Hormones also set your body's metabolism and impact your overall energy level. Lastly, hormones influence brain function—affecting your thinking ability, memory, and mood. When you consider that hormones are involved in nearly everything that goes on in your body, it's no wonder that an imbalance in hormones can cause so many health problems.

## *HormoneSynergy® for Optimal Aging*

**HormoneSynergy** refers to the interactive way that hormones influence and help each other, and emphasizes that vibrant health is the result of balanced hormones. Because hormones influence each other, one hormone out of balance can lead to imbalances of other hormones. Very low cholesterol levels can also lead to hormone imbalance, since all steroid hormones (estrogens, progesterone, testosterone, DHEA, and cortisol) have a cholesterol backbone.

Hormone balance requires adherence to the Golden Mean advocated by Aristotle—or the "Goldilocks Principle" of the fairy tale—not too much, not too little, just the right amount! This is why the standard "one-size-fits-all" approach to hormone replacement often leads to negative side effects. This is also why it is useful to test your hormone levels and to work with a physician who focuses on your individual needs.

HormoneSynergy—the state of ultimate balance and cooperation between your body's hormones—is necessary to achieve vibrant health and optimal aging. As we continue on our hormone journey, consider the following 5 HormoneSynergy Principles.

## *The 5 HormoneSynergy Principles*

1. Hormone imbalance can occur at any age, and many hormones decline with age.
2. Aging accelerates as hormone levels decline.
3. As hormone levels decline, health declines.
4. Hormone balance is greatly influenced by diet and lifestyle choices.
5. Bioidentical hormones are best if supplementing.

No matter what the term "anti-aging" implies, we all know that aging isn't optional. However, you <u>can</u> choose to experience optimal aging. Optimal aging means you can slow the effects of aging, keep your mind sharp, maintain an attractive body, and continue to experience all the joys of life. Achieving and maintaining hormone balance may also prevent chronic diseases such as diabetes, heart disease, and obesity. In addition, balanced hormones can help you avoid arthritis, osteoporosis, Alzheimer's disease and dementia, and some forms of cancer.

## Points to remember:

- Hormones are chemical messengers—they are the language cells use to communicate. For proper function, every hormone must fit its receptor exactly, like a key in a lock.

- Hormones are responsible for growth and development, and repair of the body's tissues. They also play major roles in reproduction, metabolism, and brain health. Your body requires balanced hormones in order to have healthy blood sugar regulation, immune function, and energy levels.

- Many hormones decline with age, and aging accelerates as hormones decline.

- All hormones interact with and influence one another. To experience optimal aging, your hormones must be balanced ("HormoneSynergy").

# Chapter 3: Your Traveling Companions: a Description of Your Hormones

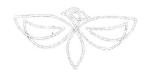

*(NB: This chapter is a reference – a mere catalog – and some readers may skip it at first, and then flip back here once they meet one of these hormones later on in the book. Feel free to do that.)*

You've already learned that hormones interact with and influence one another, and that for optimal health, all hormones must be balanced. It's now time to introduce the main hormones. Like characters in a "road trip" movie, each hormone has specific personality traits and functions. Knowing these functions will help you understand symptoms of hormone imbalance.

As you travel through life, these characters, your hormones, chatter back and forth, influencing each other and your health. All hormones are produced by glands throughout your body. Following are the glands that secrete the hormones discussed in this book:

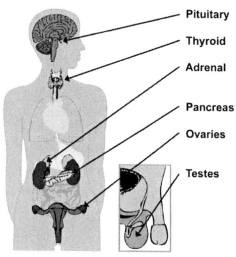

Pituitary

Thyroid

Adrenal

Pancreas

Ovaries

Testes

> **Pituitary** – makes FSH, LH, & TSH
>
> **Thyroid** – makes T4 & T3
>
> **Adrenals** – make DHEA & cortisol (and some estrogens, progesterone, & testosterone)
>
> **Pancreas** – makes insulin
>
> **Ovaries** – make estrogens, progesterone, & testosterone in women
>
> **Testes** – make testosterone in men

Next is the Cast of Characters. Meet your traveling companions.

### *Estrogen*

Estrogen is actually a collective term that refers to three main hormones: *estradiol, estrone,* and *estriol.* Estradiol is the most potent estrogen and is reversibly converted to estrone; both estradiol and estrone can be irreversibly converted to estriol.

In premenopausal women, estradiol is made by the ovaries; after menopause, estradiol is made primarily from conversion of the adrenal gland hormones DHEA and androstenedione. While estradiol is the main estrogen produced in a premenopausal woman, estrone is the main estrogen produced by fat tissue in a menopausal woman. Estriol is the weakest of the estrogens and is only made in high amounts during pregnancy.

Men also need estrogen, but in smaller amounts. The enzyme called "aromatase" is responsible for converting testosterone into estrogen in men. As men age, their estradiol level often remains the same or increases as testosterone production declines.[2] This is because aromatase activity increases with aging. Aromatase also increases when a man is overweight, since aromatase is found in high amounts in fat tissue, and in the presence of increased inflammation. High estrogen levels in men, especially coupled with low testosterone, can increase insulin resistance.[3] Insulin resistance is associated with metabolic syndrome and an increased likelihood of developing diabetes.

In women, estrogen is responsible for the development of breast tissue and reproductive organs. Although men tease each other about "man boobs," breast development in men is no laughing matter. This is a condition called "gynecomastia" and it may be a sign of high estrogen and low testosterone levels. In my work I often encounter couples where men (usually with "spare tires") have higher estrogen levels than their menopausal wives!

Healthy estrogen levels play a very important role in heart health by dilating blood vessels and increasing HDL (good) cholesterol. Estrogen also builds and preserves bone in women and men. Skin elasticity, thickness, and moisture are maintained by estrogen. This is why low estrogen levels in women can lead to wrinkles and dry skin. Adequate estrogen also ensures healthy vaginal pH to prevent infections, and normal lubrication to inhibit vaginal dryness.

One of the most crucial roles estrogen plays is in the health of your brain. Estrogen helps regenerate and preserve brain cells, and may prevent dementia and Alzheimer's.[4-7] Estrogen is also involved in learning, memory, and attention span. During menopause, declining estrogen levels contribute to memory problems and an increase in forgetfulness. Estrogen also improves mood[8] by increasing the brain's supply of "happy" molecules—serotonin, dopamine, and norepinephrine—this is why some women with declining estrogen levels become depressed or anxious.

## Points to remember about estrogen:

- Estrogen is a collective term that refers to three main estrogens: estradiol, estrone, and estriol.

- In premenopausal women, most estrogen is made by the ovaries.

- After menopause, the adrenal glands are critical for normal estrogen production.

- In men, testosterone is converted into estrogen by the aromatase enzyme (made by fat tissue and increased with inflammation and liver problems).

- Men need some estrogen, but too much can lead to breast enlargement or contribute to insulin resistance.

- Whether you are a woman or a man, you need estrogen to have a healthy heart, bones, skin, and brain.

## Progesterone

Progesterone is a hormone made by the ovaries in premenopausal women after ovulation, and by the adrenal glands in women and men. Progesterone is the precursor for production of the stress hormone, cortisol. Significant or long-term stress and high cortisol levels increase the demand for progesterone; over time, this can lead to depletion of progesterone and low levels.

In women, progesterone helps prepare for and maintain pregnancy — this is why progesterone deficiency can lead to infertility and miscarriage. Progesterone also promotes differentiation in breast cells — in other words, it makes sure that dividing breast cells become healthy, mature breast cells.

Progesterone balances estrogen in the uterus by preventing the uterine lining from getting too thick and causing heavy periods, and by inhibiting the formation of uterine fibroids and endometriosis. There is also some evidence that progesterone may help maintain bones increasing the number and maturity of osteoblasts (bone-building cells).[9,10] It may, therefore, help prevent or treat osteoporosis — although estrogen and testosterone are more important for bone building.

One of the metabolites of progesterone called "5-allopregnanolone" binds to the GABA (gamma-aminobutyric acid) receptor in the brain that promotes calmness. This is the same receptor that is affected by sleep and anxiety medications. Therefore, progesterone helps balance the stimulatory effects of estrogen in the brain, and can help with anxiety and sleep problems. In addition, progesterone often helps with PMS symptoms, such as moodiness and water weight gain.

Adequate progesterone may, theoretically, inhibit excess facial hair growth in women. This is because progesterone limits testosterone from forming its more potent metabolite dihydrotestosterone (DHT). When there's not enough progesterone to restrain it, more testosterone metabolizes into DHT, and the result may be an increase in both acne and facial hair.

## Points to remember about progesterone:

- Progesterone is made by the ovaries after ovulation in premenopausal women. The adrenal glands in both women and men make small amounts of progesterone.
- Progesterone is the precursor for stress hormones.
- Progesterone prepares for and maintains pregnancy.
- Healthy bones and breasts require adequate progesterone.
- In the uterus, progesterone balances estrogen and limits endometriosis and the formation of fibroids.
- Progesterone calms the brain.
- Optimal progesterone levels in women may help with acne and facial hair growth.

### *Testosterone*

Testosterone is often thought of as the "male" hormone. In fact testosterone is a very important hormone for both men <u>and</u> women. In men it's made primarily by the testes, and in women by the ovaries and adrenal glands.

Testosterone is an "anabolic" hormone, meaning it promotes protein synthesis for structural tissue such as muscle, bone, and the heart. Testosterone is the hormone that tells your body to build muscle. If your testosterone is low, you may find that exercising doesn't improve muscle mass, strength, or tone like it should.

Men produce significantly more testosterone than women do; this is the reason men have bigger livers, lungs, and hearts. Testosterone is critical for bone strength – it can prevent bone loss, as well as stimulate osteoblasts (bone building cells) and production of growth factors in bone. Testosterone may also prevent fractures by increasing muscle mass and strength, therefore, reducing the odds of falling and breaking a bone.

Testosterone is perhaps best known as the libido (sex drive) hormone, which is actually true for both women and men. When testosterone declines, men may experience erectile changes – fewer or absent morning erections, difficulty achieving erections, less firm erections – and sometimes difficulty having orgasms. Women with testosterone deficiency may also experience fewer or absent orgasms as well as diminished sensitivity of the clitoris.

Testosterone is very important for the health of your heart and normal blood sugar levels. Low testosterone is often associated with high insulin levels and diabetes, and testosterone supplementation can decrease insulin resistance and help prevent or reverse diabetes.[11-15] Testosterone helps maintain heart health by dilating the coronary arteries (the arteries that feed your heart), promoting normal blood pressure, and preserving strength of the heart.[16-20]

As you age, you may notice a reduction in brain function affecting your ability to learn new information or retrieve things you already know. Declining testosterone production contributes to a decreasing ability to remember words or pictures, to mentally manipulate objects in space (spatial ability), and to plan, organize, and remember details.[21] Low free testosterone levels are actually a risk factor for developing Alzheimer's disease,[22-24] which currently afflicts someone in the U.S. every 71 seconds.

In addition to improving thinking ability, testosterone facilitates the release of the neurotransmitter dopamine[25,26] — the brain chemical that enables you to concentrate or focus, and prevents depression. People with Parkinson's disease have low dopamine production and testosterone has been shown to help with Parkinson symptoms.[27-29] In addition, testosterone improves mental sharpness, memory, mood, and overall sense of well-being.

## Points to remember about testosterone:

- Testosterone is made by both men and women (men make more).
- Low testosterone may lead to decreased libido, erectile problems, and an inability to experience orgasm.
- Testosterone builds and strengthens bone and muscle.
- Testosterone protects the heart.
- Testosterone enhances insulin sensitivity and may help prevent or reverse diabetes.
- The brain needs testosterone—low levels can lead to problems with memory, an inability to focus, and depression.

## *Hormones from Your Adrenal Glands: DHEA and Cortisol*

The adrenal glands are very important in maintaining hormone balance. They have the task of making stress hormones—adrenaline and cortisol—as well as making hormones that serve as precursors for estrogens and testosterone (namely, DHEA and androstenedione). Adrenaline is a fast-acting hormone that produces a quick burst of energy, and that the body quickly eliminates. DHEA and cortisol prolong the fight-or-flight response, and also help with recovery.

Survival isn't possible without the ability to make stress hormones; however long term or chronic stress can cause or worsen many health problems and can lead to significant hormone imbalance symptoms. Chapter 4 discusses in detail how chronically elevated cortisol can lead to symptoms and health problems.

## DHEA

DHEA is the most abundant steroid hormone circulating in your body. In other words, your body makes more DHEA than it does any of the sex hormones. DHEA is a precursor for estrogen and testosterone production, especially as you age. Since DHEA does not have any direct hormone activity (in other words, it doesn't bind to specific DHEA receptors) it is mainly thought of as a "buffer" hormone, meaning it can convert into estrogens or testosterone if needed.

As you age, your DHEA production falls dramatically. This slowing down of adrenal gland output is called "adrenopause." For example, a 20-year old typically makes 30 mg of DHEA daily, whereas an 80-year old makes less than 6 mg—an 80% drop.

Many wonder if DHEA supplementation can help preserve youthfulness. Although rats don't make much DHEA to begin with, research suggests that life span and youthfulness in rats may be extended by DHEA supplementation. In humans, some studies have correlated higher DHEA levels with longer life spans.[30,31]

The age-related decline in DHEA is thought to contribute to the rise in fasting blood sugar that occurs with aging.[32] In people with high blood sugar, DHEA supplementation improves insulin sensitivity.[33]

DHEA is necessary to maintain a healthy immune system and optimal brain function. Low DHEA levels have been found in people with autoimmune diseases (especially lupus and rheumatoid arthritis), Alzheimer's disease, and dementia.[34-36] Often times the lower the DHEA, the worse the disease.

In healthy people, a low DHEA-to-cortisol ratio is common with aging and with evolving health problems.[37-40] Overall, cortisol suppresses immune function whereas DHEA supports normal immune function. Long-term stress causes the adrenal glands to shift production from DHEA to cortisol.

Like estradiol and testosterone, DHEA helps maintain healthy brain activity and prevents depression. DHEA also enhances memory by taking part in neural plasticity,[41] which allows neurons (nerve cells in the brain) to change in order to record new memories. DHEA supplementation has been shown to support glial cells, the brain cells that enhance survival of neurons.[42] In addition, DHEA actually promotes regeneration of neurons in the hippocampus,[43] an area of the brain that plays a major role in short term memory and the formation of new memory. The hippocampus is often damaged by chronic stress levels and is one of the first areas of the brain destroyed by Alzheimer's. DHEA supplementation has been shown to have antidepressant effects in the brain.[44,45]

DHEA is available as an over-the-counter supplement, but it should only be taken with proper monitoring. Excess DHEA supplementation can cause side effects and may be contraindicated with some health problems. How can DHEA be monitored? Test your DHEA-sulphate level — this is the storage form of DHEA and is less subject to fluctuations — both before and after supplementation. Make sure you work with an experienced physician to ensure that DHEA supplementation is right for you.

## Cortisol

In response to stress, the adrenal glands produce another hormone, cortisol. To the human body, cortisol is as powerful a force as the wind — small amounts can be put to good use (think sailboats and windmills), but high levels over time can be as devastating as a hurricane.

When your body's stress response is triggered — by anything — cortisol jumps in, increasing blood sugar and blood pressure. This helps to pump blood, oxygen, and fuel to your brain, muscles, and vital organs.

As your body's natural anti-inflammatory hormone, normal amounts of cortisol keep inflammation under control. You may be familiar with a group of anti-inflammatory medications called "corticosteroids." The corticosteroids are similar to cortisol in their function; they are powerful drugs used in asthma inhalers and to suppress dangerous allergic responses and the symptoms of autoimmune diseases. Keeping your body's own production of cortisol in balance is crucial for balanced immune function.

During the stress response, cortisol enables your brain to adapt to a changing environment by increasing production of the neurotransmitter (or brain chemical) called *glutamate*. Glutamate is necessary for thinking, learning, and memory. However, too much glutamate can cause shrinking of brain cells and even brain cell death (more on this in chapter 4).

## Points to remember about adrenal gland hormones:

- The adrenal glands make stress hormones (adrenaline and cortisol), DHEA, progesterone, and precursors for estrogen and testosterone.

- Stress hormones produced by the adrenal glands are necessary for survival.

- Chronic stress can lead to an imbalance in adrenal gland hormones, followed by a breakdown of health and rapid aging.

### *Thyroid hormones*

The thyroid gland produces two hormones (T4 and T3) that control body development, growth, and metabolism. More than 90% of the hormones secreted by the thyroid is T4 (thyroxine); however, T4 is mostly inactive. To become active, T4 must be converted by the body into its active form, T3 (triiodothyronine). Regulation of thyroid hormone is controlled by the brain (via the hypothalamus and pituitary), the thyroid gland itself, and peripheral conversion of inactive T4 into active T3. Therefore, low thyroid (hypothyroid) symptoms can result from multiple causes:

- a problem in the brain
- a problem in the thyroid gland
- poor conversion of thyroid hormone from T4 into T3

Thyroid hormone is needed by every cell of your body. Without it, cells cannot function normally—this is why thyroid hormone deficiency can cause problems in every body system. Thyroid hormone is the main hormone responsible for metabolism and energy levels. It's also critical for normal immune function, as well as healthy skin, hair, and nails.

Thyroid hormone is essential for contraction of your heart; low thyroid hormone level ("hypothyroidism") can cause heart enlargement and low pulse rate. Hypothyroidism can also cause high LDL ("bad") cholesterol, the type of cholesterol that can become oxidized, leading to plaques in the arteries.

Muscles require thyroid hormone for strength and function—in fact, a low thyroid hormone level is commonly associated with muscle aching or weakness.

Lastly, thyroid hormone is vital for the health of your brain—it maintains a positive, stable mood and improves the speed of thinking. Without enough thyroid hormone, you can become depressed or anxious. This is in part due to T3 (active thyroid hormone) working between neurons to regulate the amount and activity of neurotransmitters (brain chemicals) such as serotonin and GABA.[46,47]

## Points to remember about thyroid hormone

- Comes in two types:
  - o T4 (inactive thyroid hormone) is
    - produced by the thyroid gland and
    - converted to T3 (active thyroid hormone) throughout the body
  - o T3 (active thyroid hormone)
- Needed by every cell of the body
- Necessary for healthy skin, hair, and nails
- Essential for normal immune function
- Required for the contraction of the heart and normal cholesterol levels
- Needed by muscles for strength and function
- Supports healthy brain function and mood

## Insulin

Insulin was the first hormone identified (in the 1920s), which won Dr. Frederick Banting and his medical student, Charles Best, the Nobel Prize. As with stress hormones, human life is not possible without insulin. Insulin is made by the pancreas, and is released in response to the amount of glucose (sugar) in your bloodstream. Insulin's main job is to enable your body's cells to take up glucose. Cells can use the glucose for immediate fuel, or fat cells can store it for later use. Your liver and muscles can also convert glucose to glycogen (a more temporary storage form than fat).

Your abdomen contains a lot of insulin receptors; this is why high insulin levels can lead to weight gain around your waist.

There are two main diseases associated with insulin production. Both are called "diabetes" though they originate differently. The first, the inability to make enough insulin, is referred to as "type 1" diabetes. The second, making too much insulin, is referred to as "type 2" diabetes.

Unmanaged diabetes increases the risk for heart attack, stroke, kidney failure, blindness, Alzheimer's disease, cancer, and amputations.

Type 2 diabetes accounts for 90 to 95 percent of all diabetes cases. Type 2 diabetes is preceded by two other conditions: "insulin resistance" and "impaired fasting glucose." Both of these conditions are nearly always preventable and reversible.

*Insulin resistance* is a condition where cells ignore normal levels of insulin, and the pancreas must generate larger and larger amounts of insulin to lower glucose in the bloodstream. Cells become resistant to the excessive amounts of insulin, leaving more and more sugar in the blood.

*Impaired fasting glucose* is a condition where a person's blood contains an unusually high amount of sugar, even after they've gone without eating for several hours.

Among all US adults, nearly 26% currently have impaired fasting glucose and insulin resistance, often thought of as pre-diabetes. In this age group, nearly 11% have diabetes. Among people over 60, the percentage of diabetics jumps to 23%. This means that more than 80 million Americans are currently insulin resistant or have type 2 diabetes.[48]

Insulin resistance occurs in a step-wise fashion: initially, high blood sugar (from eating too many refined carbohydrates or long-term stress) causes the pancreas to secrete excessive amounts of insulin. If this continues, eventually cells won't respond to the high level of insulin—they become resistant.

Insulin resistance by cells is similar to what would happen if someone who'd visited too often continues to knock on your door—you start to ignore them. The pancreas responds to the high blood sugar by making even more insulin (the knocking continues and gets louder). When the pancreas cannot make enough insulin to bring down blood sugar, the blood sugar stays high. If fasting blood sugar is >126 mg/dL, a person now meets the diagnostic criteria for type 2 diabetes.

As you can see, type 2 diabetes doesn't happen overnight—there are many options to reverse insulin resistance, including exercise, diet and lifestyle changes, nutrient supplementation, and maintaining optimal hormone levels (discussed in chapter 6). Even if you have a strong family history of diabetes, the Nurses' Health Study suggests that 90% of type 2 diabetes can be attributed to four factors within your control: excess weight, lack of exercise, poor diet, and smoking.[49] Remember, you are not your genes—you are how your genes express themselves.

Whether or not you have diabetes, high insulin levels are dangerous and disruptive to all other hormones and body systems. High insulin accelerates aging and leads to chronic inflammation and degenerative disease.

We can learn a lot about how to age optimally by studying centenarians—people who live to be 100 yrs old. Only 1 in 10,000 people in the US will become a centenarian; therefore, adopting the following habits common to people who've celebrated their 100th birthday may improve your odds:

- don't develop insulin resistance or diabetes
- don't eat too many calories
- consume a lot of antioxidants and plant foods to prevent "internal rusting"
- maintain high HDL ("good") cholesterol levels by eating well and exercising

**Points to remember about insulin:**

- Insulin is made by the pancreas in response to blood sugar.
- If blood sugar is repeatedly high, insulin resistance can develop; this is the precursor to type 2 diabetes.
- Too much insulin increases fat storage, especially around the waist.
- High insulin disrupts all other hormones, accelerates aging, promotes chronic inflammation, and contributes to degenerative diseases.

## *Vitamin D*

You may be surprised to see a vitamin included in a chapter about hormones, however, active vitamin D is actually a hormone. Vitamin D receptors have been found in the brain, heart, skin, and white blood cells. The reproductive organs such as the ovaries, breasts, testes, and prostate gland also contain vitamin D receptors.

Vitamin D performs several functions in your body. It has long been known that vitamin D regulates calcium and phosphorous in the bloodstream and promotes bone formation and mineralization. New research is revealing the role vitamin D plays in the immune system. For example, vitamin D enhances *phagocytosis*, a process by which certain white blood cells engulf bacteria, dead cells, and other debris. Vitamin D also plays a role in preventing autoimmune diseases. Low vitamin D has been associated with rheumatoid arthritis, lupus, Crohn's disease, ulcerative colitis, multiple sclerosis, psoriasis, and fibromyalgia. People who suffer from muscle and chronic pain, psoriasis, heart disease, and breast, prostate, and colon cancers are also more likely to have low vitamin D levels.

Perhaps the most exciting research about vitamin D is its ability to prevent some cancers. Vitamin D appears to play a role in cell proliferation (division) and differentiation (making sure dividing cells don't become cancerous cells). In addition, vitamin D is involved in proper death of unhealthy or old cells, a process known as "apoptosis," and in the prevention of blood vessel formation to feed existing cancers, known as "angiogenesis."[50,51]

The first randomized, placebo-controlled trial evaluating vitamin D supplementation and the incidence of cancer was published, in 2007 — in that study, women using 1100 IU of vitamin $D_3$ daily for 4 years had a 60% lower cancer risk than the placebo group. When patients who were diagnosed with cancer during the first year of the study were excluded (with the assumption that they likely had cancer when they entered the study), the reduction was 77%.[52] This is exciting news since there aren't many supplements that have been shown to lower cancer risk by such a large margin.

Vitamin D is also an important anti-aging hormone since it actually slows the shortening of your telomeres[53] — the end segments of chromosomes that protect your DNA. Optimal vitamin D levels are thought to slow your speed of aging by at least 5 years.

Your skin makes vitamin D from exposure to the sun. As you age, however, your skin becomes less able to make vitamin D. When taking vitamin D, it's important to measure and monitor vitamin D levels closely. Too much vitamin D can cause calcification of soft tissues and an increased risk of kidney stones. It's especially important to monitor your levels if you are supplementing with doses greater than 2,000 IU of $D_3$ per day. Chapter 4 provides more information about vitamin D testing.

**Points to remember about vitamin D:**

- Active vitamin D is a hormone.
- Vitamin D is involved in the health of many organs and glands — receptors for vitamin D have been found in the brain, heart, skin, white blood cells, ovaries, breasts, testes, and the prostate.
- Vitamin D plays a role in promoting healthy bones.
- Optimal vitamin D levels ensure a healthy immune system and may prevent autoimmune diseases and some cancers.

# Chapter 4: Symptoms of Hormone Imbalance

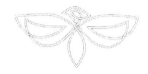

You've met the cast of characters — now we hit the road. Here are the symptoms you, your family, or friends may be experiencing on your health journey, and what can cause each of them.

### Estrogen Dominance

Women may experience hormone imbalance symptoms at any age. Starting with the onset of menses, an imbalance in the ratio between estrogen and progesterone can cause symptoms often referred to as "estrogen dominance" — meaning too much estrogen relative to progesterone.

Kari, a 39-year-old mother and hair stylist, struggled significantly with estrogen dominance. Here was Kari's story during her initial visit:

> I've had problems with my period off and on throughout my life. In fact, it took many months to get pregnant with each of my kids. Over the past several cycles my periods have been really heavy, and the cramps during the first few days are so severe, even ibuprofen doesn't help. Also, I have to admit, my mood is so up and down before my period. I find myself crying at commercials one minute, and yelling at my husband the next.

When I asked Kari if she noticed any cravings or changes in her weight she confided:

> Oh, yes, I've gained 25 pounds over the past couple of years from eating too many carbs — as many bagels, scones, and chocolate as I can get my hands on. I really feel out of control about it. I'm also drinking more than I used to — 2 or 3 glasses of wine every night.

As in Kari's case, estrogen dominance can lead to PMS (or "premenstrual syndrome") symptoms such as mood swings, irritability, or weepiness. Many women also experience food cravings, especially simple carbohydrates, chocolate, or sweets. These symptoms may also be related to serotonin insufficiency, which in turn is often caused by chronic stress.

In addition to PMS, estrogen dominance or inadequate progesterone can lead to anxiety and sleep problems. Some women with estrogen dominance have bloating and water weight gain, as well as breast tenderness or fibrocystic breast changes before their period.

Progesterone opposes the stimulating influence of estrogen on the uterine lining. When progesterone is overwhelmed by estrogen dominance, the result can be prolonged or heavy periods, or significant menstrual cramps. Too much estrogen stimulation can also cause uterine fibroids to develop and grow.

Estrogen dominance symptoms can be caused by five main problems:

- Too much estrogen production
- Inability to eliminate estrogen from the body
- Exposure to xenoestrogens
- Lack of ovulation
- High stress levels

## Too much estrogen production

First off, many women produce too much estrogen from being overweight. This is because the aromatase enzyme increases with fat tissue. Aromatase converts hormone precursors, such as testosterone, androstenedione, and DHEA, into estrogen. In Kari's case, extra body fat contributed to her symptoms of estrogen dominance.

## Inability to eliminate estrogen from the body

The second cause of estrogen dominance is the inability to effectively metabolize and excrete estrogens. This can be due to constipation or poor liver function. Normally, estrogens are conjugated in the liver and excreted into the intestines via bile. Constipation can enable intestinal bacteria to deconjugate the excreted estrogens, allowing them to be reabsorbed and recirculated throughout the body (this phenomenon is known as "enterohepatic circulation"). This unhealthy recirculation of estrogen is worse if a woman lacks    adequate beneficial bacteria,[54] such as *Lactobacillus* and *Bifidobacterium.* Similarly, poor liver function from genetics or the liver being overwhelmed by toxicity, can cause estrogen to be continually recirculated. Kari's estrogen dominance symptoms were exacerbated by working in a hair salon and drinking excessive amounts of alcohol. Her liver was too overwhelmed with toxins to effectively metabolize and excrete the estrogens in her body. Kari went through a detox program, avoiding as many toxins as possible while supporting her liver by taking certain supplements. This detox regimen played a crucial role in returning her to hormone balance.

## Exposure to xenoestrogens

The third cause of estrogen dominance is excess exposure to "xenoestrogens" — synthetic chemicals in the environment that mimic estrogen in the body. Although these foreign estrogen-like molecules are weak in activity, the excessive amounts of them in the environment can overwhelm the body's ability to excrete them. In Kari's case, we discovered she had significant amounts of bisphenol-A in her body due to drinking water from plastic bottles. Research has shown that BPA levels increase substantially from drinking out of plastic bottles after only one week.[55]  Fortunately, Kari now drinks from glass containers or uses a "BPA-free" water bottle during the day. Chapter 6 includes a list of xenoestrogens, and what you can do to support your body's detoxification system.

## Lack of ovulation

The fourth cause of estrogen dominance is lack of ovulation. Although small amounts of progesterone are made in the adrenal glands, most is made by the ovary after ovulation has occurred. Each time the ovary doesn't ovulate as expected, it also doesn't produce progesterone. As women approach menopause, it becomes very common to experience cycles where no ovulation occurs. These "anovulatory cycles" can lead to shorter or longer cycles, heavier bleeding, and increased size of uterine fibroids. Kari's ovaries probably didn't ovulate every month, which was part of her problem getting pregnant and caused her irregular cycles. The herb, *Vitex agnus-castus,* or chaste tree berry can be helpful in enhancing ovulation in women as well as treating PMS symptoms.[56,57]

## High stress levels

The last main reason for estrogen dominance is long-term, high levels of stress. This is because the adrenal glands convert progesterone into cortisol—short-term survival is more important to the body than balanced reproductive hormones. When stress stretches out over a long time, the body continues to convert progesterone into cortisol, leaving a progesterone deficiency that contributes to estrogen dominance symptoms. In Kari's case, after we discussed the relationship between her symptoms and stress level, she decided to commit to "emptying her stress bucket" every day. She started prioritizing sleep, attending regular yoga classes, and learned to say no to extra projects or demands when she felt over-extended. These simple changes were powerful medicine in Kari's journey to hormone balance.

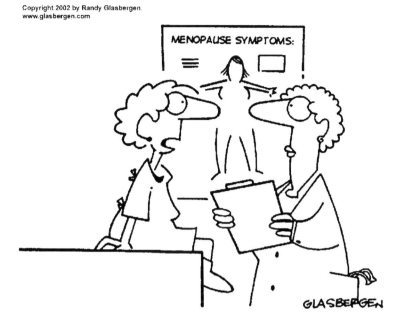

"**Frankly, I wouldn't mind the insomnia at all
if I hadn't lost my libido at the same time!**"

## *Perimenopause and Menopause*

As women age, declining estrogen, progesterone, and testosterone production may lead to many different symptoms. Before periods stop, there is a time of fluctuating hormone levels. This time, called perimenopause, can last anywhere from one to ten or more years before menopause. Menopause is defined as beginning one year after a woman stops having periods.

Diane was 51 years old when she first came in for help with perimenopausal symptoms. She looked exhausted, frazzled, and frustrated, especially since she'd gotten lost on the way to my office. Before even sitting down she pleaded:

> *I just don't know what to do anymore. I've seen my primary care doctor at least five times over the past year. All he does is tell me to take antidepressants and sleeping pills, and learn to live with my symptoms because they're a normal part of aging – "It's just menopause," he says, "you'll get through it." Well, I haven't slept in over a year. I wake up sweating all night long, throw the covers*

*off, finally fall back asleep, then wake up again freezing cold. I'm totally exhausted. During the day, I'll be in a meeting and I can feel the heat extending up my neck to my face. It's so embarrassing.*

Diane was experiencing the most recognized symptoms of menopause—hot flashes and night sweats, known in the medical world as "vasomotor symptoms." Hot flashes may be preceded by heart palpitations or heart racing, and feelings of anxiety—many women even describe hot flashes being accompanied by a sense of "impending doom." Hot flashes and night sweats are more severe and frequent with stress. At least one third of women experience such severe hot flashes that their sleep and daily life are significantly affected.

Sleep problems are very common during menopause. Problems falling asleep or staying asleep may or may not be related to hot flashes or night sweats. Many women notice that when their estrogen is low, they can't sleep well no matter what they do. In some women with low estrogen, all the usual treatments—lowering stress, using natural sleep aids, or taking sleep medications—may be ineffective. This type of insomnia can often be eliminated with bioidentical estrogen or testosterone supplementation.

During her menopausal transition, Susan, a 53-year old attorney, experienced milder hot flashes than Diane. Her biggest concern was a decline in thinking ability and fear of dementia. Here's Susan's story:

*I can live with hot flashes and changes in my appearance, but I can't deal with the changes in my brain. It's like I'm going crazy. I've always been sharp, focused, articulate. I'm an accomplished woman in my field. Lately, I feel like I'm hiding what's going on inside. I find myself in the middle of a sentence and I can't remember what I was about to say. Other times I'll be reading and I get lost in the middle of a paragraph. I've even been driving when all of a sudden I can't remember where I'm going. I also get anxious in situations that didn't use to faze me—the other day I felt like I was going to have a panic attack. I've never had anxiety in my life and I feel like I've lost my self-confidence. I'm really concerned about all of this—my mother has dementia and I'm terrified of losing my mind.*

As discussed earlier, estrogen and testosterone are very important hormones for the brain. As Susan's hormones declined, she, like many women, experienced memory problems and foggy thinking. Women often describe words "vanishing" while they're talking, or that they can't remember experiences that happened recently. Depression and anxiety are common since estrogen and testosterone are needed for optimal serotonin and dopamine levels in the brain. Some women struggle with emotional mood swings and increased irritability, sometimes describing themselves as "not feeling very loving" toward family or people in general.

Carol's story is unique, since her skin is important for her ability to make a living. Before she achieved hormone balance, she described her appearance this way:

> *I don't mean to be vain, but I own a popular salon in town and people judge me by my appearance. I used to get comments that I looked 10 or 20 years younger than my age. Since turning 60, nobody mistakes me for 40 anymore! I use the most advanced anti-aging skin care line available, which does help some. But my skin is so loose now, it just sags in places. I see pictures of myself and I look old. I just can't believe how fast my skin has aged.*

When I asked Carol about other menopause related symptoms, she admitted:

> *My hair is definitely thinner than it used to be. In fact, I feel like twice as much falls out as grows in. Vaginal dryness? It's like sandpaper down there. Anyway, that doesn't really bother me since I have absolutely no sex drive.*

Carol knew firsthand how important estrogen is for  promoting normal collagen and elastin formation. These proteins are essential for keeping skin strong, supple, and elastic. Declining estrogen often leads to wrinkles, thinning skin, easy bruising, and atrophy (thinning) of the vaginal canal. Estrogen and testosterone enhance lubrication preventing skin, hair, and vaginal tissue from becoming dry. As the lining of the vaginal canal becomes thinner and dryer, leakage of urine can occur, as well as an increased risk for developing urinary tract and vaginal infections.

Many symptoms familiar to menopausal women are actually related, not just to low estrogen, but to decreased production of testosterone. In fact, most tissues that have estrogen receptors also make aromatase, the enzyme that converts testosterone into estrogen.[58,59] This means that the brain, bones, heart, blood vessels, and skin can all produce estrogen from testosterone.

By age 40, women produce approximately half the testosterone they did in their 20s (although estrogen production is usually still quite high).[60,61] Women may notice symptoms related to declining testosterone similar to Sharon, a 42-year-old business owner, who came in with these concerns:

> *I've started slowing down recently, like I don't have the energy to do all the things I used to do. For most of my life I've enjoyed going for a run in the morning and working out at the gym. Now it seems like I've lost my motivation, it's like a chore to exercise. I also don't feel as strong as I did. It takes me several days to recover when I do exercise, and I usually wake up stiff and sore. Also, I've been gaining weight lately even though my eating hasn't changed.*

Sharon's symptoms were mainly due to decreased testosterone levels. In women, low testosterone commonly leads to fatigue and poor stamina since adequate testosterone is needed for energy production. Testosterone is also essential to build structural tissue, which is the reason testosterone deficiency can lead to reduced lean body mass— meaning more fat, less muscle, and decreased bone formation.[62] Testosterone enhances joint lubrication and inhibits inflammation;[63,64] insufficient levels can lead to increased joint pain and stiffness, especially in the morning (similar to a "creaky gate").

As seen in Diane's case, both testosterone and estrogen are needed by the brain. Low testosterone can lead to difficulty concentrating and focusing, as well as a decreased sense of well-being, depression, and memory problems.

Without adequate testosterone production, a woman's libido can drop and may even fade away completely. With low testosterone, some women have decreased sensitivity in their clitoris and may become unable to experience orgasm. Debra, a vibrant 57-year-old woman, describes it this way:

> *My husband and I have been married for more than 30 years. I've always felt great about our love life. Some of my friends complain about their husbands but I've always been grateful that Jim and I could connect through being intimate. You can imagine how devastated I was when my libido disappeared in my mid 40s and I couldn't have orgasms anymore. At first I thought there was*

*something wrong with me or with my marriage — we went to couples' counseling and even went to a sex therapist. When I found out my testosterone level was basically zero and Dr. Retzler treated me with bioidentical testosterone pellets, I was so relieved. I'm happy to report my husband and I have our passion back!*

Although it's often overlooked, testosterone truly is a crucial hormone for women.

As women age and go through menopause, the adrenal glands take over the role the ovaries performed earlier in life. It's very important that women transition into menopause with healthy adrenal gland function to minimize menopausal symptoms. In postmenopausal women the adrenal glands make androstenedione and DHEA (which are converted into estrogens and testosterone) and progesterone. Chronic stress can diminish the adrenal glands' ability to take on this function. If the adrenal glands are struggling to keep up with a high demand for stress hormones, they may not be able to produce enough estrogen, progesterone, or testosterone, making menopausal symptoms worse. Most peri and postmenopausal women will agree — hormone imbalance symptoms worsen during times of increased stress.

Following are symptoms associated with perimenopause and menopause:

- Menstrual irregularities
- Hot flashes
- Night sweats
- Heart palpitations
- Headaches
- Poor sleep
- Irritability
- Mood swings
- Foggy thinking
- Decreased concentration or focus
- Blunted motivation
- Memory problems
- Depression or anxiety
- Vaginal dryness
- Painful intercourse
- Urinary tract infections
- Breast tenderness
- Thinning skin or wrinkles
- Increased facial hair
- Joint stiffness or pain

- Fat accumulation
- Decreased muscle tone and mass
- Low bone density
- Hair loss
- Fatigue

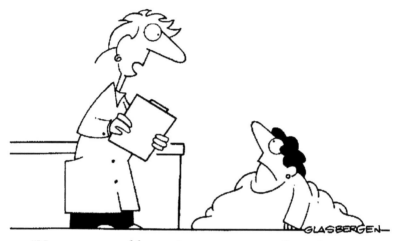

**"Menopause and low estrogen can cause bone loss...
but usually it's slower and less severe."**

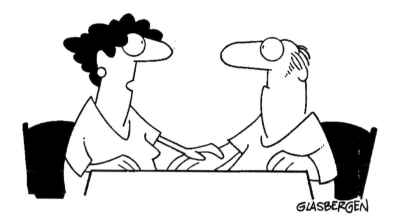

"You and I make a great team. But I wish we'd score more often!"

## Andropause: the Male Menopause

Ask the average guy what he knows about hormones and he might say "Hormones are the reason women get all emotional before their period" or "Hormones are why women have hot flashes and get crabby when they go through menopause." Many men don't realize the crucial role hormones play in their own bodies — or recognize that hormone imbalance, such as declining testosterone levels, can cause significant and progressive symptoms in men.

The term "andropause" is often referred to as "male menopause." The medical community acknowledges the existence of "androgen decline in the aging male," a.k.a. "ADAM," although not all physicians agree that low testosterone levels in aging men should be treated. Symptoms of andropause usually come on gradually due to the slow, steady nature of the decline in testosterone, often coupled with an increase in estrogen production.

Unfortunately, testosterone production in American men has been declining for more than two decades.[65] For example, in 1988, 50-year-old men had higher testosterone levels than 50-year-old men in 1996. The reasons for this decline are unclear; however, neither aging nor other health factors such as obesity or smoking, completely explain the decline. It's likely that certain environmental toxins play a role in this phenomenon (see "Step 5" in chapter 6 for more on environmental toxicity). Low testosterone levels are commonly seen in men over age 40, with levels decreasing as early as the 30s. Recent studies suggest the prevalence of low testosterone in men over 35 years may be as high as 38.7%,[66] with >50% of men having low testosterone by age 80.[67] Inadequate testosterone production may be even more common; for example, if the diagnosis is based on free testosterone levels (the amount that's available to the body's tissues), many more men would meet the criteria for low testosterone.

As a result of aging, there are three main causes of low testosterone in men:

- Decreased testosterone production in the testes
- Increased level of testosterone-absorbing sex hormone binding globulin (SHBG)
- Elevated level of aromatase, converting testosterone into estrogens

Decreased testosterone production from the testes is the primary cause of age-related testosterone decline.

Another contributing factor is increased production of the testosterone-binding protein called "sex hormone binding globulin (SHBG)." SHBG is like a sponge, soaking up testosterone so less is available to the body's tissues.

A third contributing factor to andropause is an elevated amount of aromatase—the enzyme that converts testosterone to estrogens. Aromatase levels rise with fat tissue, inflammation, and aging. Therefore, as men age, gain weight, or produce high amounts of inflammation, their testosterone levels may plummet while estrogen levels surge.

Symptoms of andropause are numerous, including increased fat deposition, especially around the waist (often called a "spare tire"), and decreased muscle mass and strength. Richard had a classic case of andropause-induced weight gain when he came to see me at age 58.

Richard was 6 feet tall and his weight had climbed from 170 lbs in his 20s, to 245 lbs in his 50s. Not only did he have a "spare tire" but he started noticing an increase in the breast area. As Richard put it:

*I guess I just need to hit the gym harder. As it is, I meet with a personal trainer 3 days a week and I play basketball on the weekends. I realize I've gained some weight but I didn't know I was technically obese. Since my dad had a heart attack around my age, I'm worried about my high cholesterol and blood sugar. It just seems harder and harder to exercise — frankly, I'm exhausted by the time I get home from work.*

Low testosterone can cause a vicious cycle of weight gain — testosterone deficiency reduces muscle mass and increases fat, then the excess fat raises aromatase levels. The additional aromatase converts more testosterone to estrogens, in turn furthering fat accumulation. In addition, high estrogen production in men may worsen insulin resistance, often accompanied by weight gain.

As testosterone declines, men often notice joint stiffness or pain. Muscle loss, aching, and weakness from testosterone deficiency are often chalked up to laziness or being out of shape.

Mike had been dismissing his andropause symptoms for years before his wife pressured him to see me. As a retired firefighter, Mike had a history of dealing with his own symptoms privately, including his exhaustion and worsening joint and muscle pain. After lab work showed Mike his symptoms weren't "all in his head," but were due to severe testosterone deficiency and anemia, Mike related how bad he'd really been feeling:

*When I was young, I remember having so much energy. I loved being a firefighter because of the physical fitness required, and the challenge of working 24-hour shifts. When I look back, I guess I started going downhill in my 40s. By the time I reached 50, I knew I had to retire. Every day I woke up in pain — I seemed to hurt all over, joints, muscles, you name it. My doctor said I had fibromyalgia and gave me painkillers and an antidepressant. I just didn't want to start taking all that stuff.*

Mike's reluctance to take medications for his symptoms enabled him to be open to new information and, eventually, to treat the cause. When Mike restored his testosterone to youthful levels, his energy improved and over time, his pain diminished.

Besides preventing weight gain and muscle and joint pain, testosterone helps build bone and increases erythropoietin, the hormone that stimulates the bone marrow to make red blood cells. In some men, significantly decreased testosterone production can lead to osteoporosis and anemia.

It's very common for low testosterone to cause fatigue and poor stamina in men. Some men will also experience a depressed mood, irritability, and apathy— just wanting to lie on the couch and watch TV. Declining testosterone levels can lead to a lack of motivation and ambition—some men describe it as a "loss of a competitive edge." Unfortunately, symptoms of low testosterone are often dismissed as signs of "just getting older."

Dan suspected his testosterone was low when he came to see me several years ago. He'd been reading about his symptoms on the Internet and recognized a change in his mental function. As the CEO of a large corporation, Dan knew he needed help when he found himself unable to keep up in his work:

> *I'm the least lazy person I know. I still get up at 6:00 am for work every day, and I really do love my job. But honestly, I don't have the same drive I used to — I just don't have the same motivation to succeed. I also notice that I'm not as creative with problem solving. As far as my mood, I think it's fine but my wife says I'm irritable and I have a short-fuse with my sons. She's also worried that I don't want to do the things I used to, like golfing on the weekends.*

Since testosterone is essential for the brain, testosterone deficiency can cause memory problems, poor concentration and focus, and lower productivity; this prevents many men, like Dan, from achieving a high level of performance in work or athletic endeavors.

Testosterone is perhaps best known for promoting a robust libido (sex drive) as well as normal erectile function. It would seem that millions of men suffer from a "Viagra® deficiency" with all the emphasis on taking medications that improve erection. Although it's not always considered, the problem may be low testosterone,[68] and testosterone supplementation may actually reverse erectile dysfunction.[69,70] Andropause-related erectile problems include decreased morning erections and the inability to achieve or maintain erections. Besides testosterone deficiency, erectile dysfunction may be due to diabetes, high blood pressure, arteriosclerosis, psychological concerns, or medication side effects. When testosterone levels decline, men may also experience a decreased volume of ejaculate or semen.

Besides producing andropause symptoms, testosterone deficiency has been linked to many health abnormalities and diseases. For example, low testosterone is associated with increased body mass index and waist-to-hip ratio (meaning an expanding waistline).[71] Testosterone deficiency is also associated with decreased HDL (good) cholesterol and increased LDL (bad) cholesterol, as well as increased insulin levels and diabetes.[72-75]  Other symptoms linked to low testosterone include high blood pressure and excess fibrinogen, a sticky protein that forms blood clots when activated.[76,77]  Men with low testosterone levels are, therefore, at an increased risk for several diseases common with aging—specifically, Alzheimer's, diabetes, heart disease and stroke.

The following symptoms and conditions may be associated with low or declining testosterone production:

- Rapid aging
- Weight gain, especially around the middle
- Decreased muscle mass and strength
- Fatigue
- Poor stamina
- Lack of motivation
- Depression
- Low libido
- Erectile dysfunction
- Joint pain or stiffness
- High blood sugar and diabetes
- Heart disease
- Alzheimer's disease
- Fibromyalgia
- Anemia
- Osteoporosis

### Adrenal Excess & Fatigue

We've repeatedly noted the hormonal imbalances and damage related to excessive stress. So, what exactly is stress? Simply put, stress is any change to which your body must adapt. The feelings and symptoms of stress are due to a sequence of biochemical events in your body, collectively called the "stress response."

The stress response is controlled by your nervous system—which is the immediate, fight-or-flight part—and your endocrine system, which makes stress hormones. During the initial phases of stress or if stress is short-term, your adrenal glands produce adrenaline and cortisol to support the physical demands that may be necessary for survival. Over time, however, excess stress hormones can damage your health. If stress levels are high enough and continue long enough, the adrenal glands can become exhausted. This condition is described as "adrenal burnout" or "adrenal fatigue."

Remember that, in the short term, the stress response is a way to prioritize some body functions while limiting others. It is designed to save your life when you're threatened. When the stress response is triggered, your heart rate, blood pressure, and blood sugar increase to pump more oxygen and fuel to your brain and muscles. As blood flow is increased to the brain and muscles, it is taken away from internal organs, particularly the organs of the digestive tract. Knowing your body's normal responses to stress will enable you to understand the digestive problems that can result when the stress response is triggered.

Ron, a 33-year-old husband, father, and commercial real estate broker, was unaware of the effects of stress on his digestive system when he first came to my clinic. He explained:

> *My main concern is irritable bowel syndrome — I've got a lot of pain, gas, diarrhea, sometimes a little nausea, that sort of thing. It doesn't seem to matter what I eat. I've eliminated wheat, dairy, and all sugar in the past trying to find out what's causing the symptoms.*

When I asked Ron about his stress level and where he ate his meals, he replied:

> *The main stress in my life is my work — with the economy down, I'm constantly worried about closing any deals. I usually skip breakfast, or grab Starbucks and a bagel, lunch is at my desk or on the road, and I often eat dinner when I get home around 8 pm.*

Ron's symptoms noticeably improved when he learned that, every time his body triggered a stress response, the "rest and digest" part of his nervous system was turned off. During or following a stressful event, you may experience familiar symptoms such as heartburn, nausea, gas, bloating, diarrhea, or constipation. Once the stress event passes, your body should return to normal. When stress is chronic, however, your body's alarm response stays on. This can lead to chronic digestive problems, as in Ron's case. It can also cause high blood pressure and elevated blood sugar. If blood sugar remains high long enough, insulin resistance, weight gain, and diabetes can result.

Chronic stress can also negatively affect the immune system, as in the case of Lisa, a 43-year-old working mom, who was also taking care of her own mother. Lisa sought help because she was tired, depressed, gaining weight, and had trouble getting out of bed in the morning. In fact, Lisa mentioned she found herself in tears often, wondering how she could keep going. She experienced frequent infections and body aches, and wondered if she had an underlying serious disease. "I think there's something wrong with my immune system," she worried, "at least once a month I have a cold, sore throat, or the flu. I feel like I hardly have a chance to get better before I get sick again. And my body aches especially at night, like my bones and joints hurt."

When I asked Lisa to take me through a typical day for her, she explained:

> Well, I drag myself out of bed at 6:00 to get the kids ready for school. I run on the treadmill for 30 minutes, take the dog for a quick walk, shower, and rush off to work. I'm an assistant for a very successful executive. I like my job, but it's extremely demanding. I'm at the office by 8:00 am – after work I go home and make dinner. My mother also lives with us. She's got severe rheumatoid arthritis and is in a lot of pain most of the time. I take her to doctors' appointments and church functions because she can't drive. Anyway, after dinner I help the kids with their homework and get ready for the next day. I'm in bed by 10:30 most nights, but I have trouble falling asleep and I wake up for at least an hour around 2:00 or 3:00 am. Sometimes I don't ever get back to sleep.

I asked Lisa when she had time for herself, time to unwind without responsibility or demands. She looked at me like I was crazy:

> I don't know what that even means. My phone is always ringing – somebody always needs something – my boss, my kids, my husband, my mother. On weekends I barely catch up on laundry or my "to do" list.

Lisa's lab work showed that she didn't have any serious illness or immune dysfunction, but her body was flooded with stress hormones all day long. Her high levels of stress hormones prevented her from falling asleep when she went to bed, and even woke her up in the middle of the night. Lisa's frequent colds and infections were an indication that her immune system couldn't respond like it should; and her lack of sleep prevented her body from repairing itself.

Lisa was relieved to understand that her health problems could be reversed by getting a handle on her stress. Lisa now knows that the stress response is like a switch that should only be flipped when needed, not every day, all day long. Frequent triggering of the stress response led to her immune dysfunction, increased inflammation, and pain.

Hyper-immune responses, such as allergies and autoimmune diseases, can also develop with chronic stress. Immune suppression, as in Lisa's case, can increase the risk for frequent infections and even, cancer. This is, in part, because chronic stress suppresses natural killer function.[78,79] Natural killer cells are part of your body's surveillance system — their job is to circulate and destroy cancerous and viral-infected cells. A meta-analysis published in 2004 reviewing more than 300 studies regarding stress and the immune system concluded that chronic stress suppresses all aspects of immunity,[80] increasing the risk for repeated infections and cancer.

High stress hormones can also lead to other hormone imbalances. For example, cortisol suppresses growth hormone — a pituitary hormone responsible for growth during childhood, and repair of tissues and slowed aging in adulthood. When growth hormone is suppressed, as it was in Lisa's case due to her lack of sleep, wounds and injuries may heal slowly. Children can actually stop growing (a condition called "stress dwarfism") with severe stress, and adults may experience rapid aging (recall the rapidly aging faces of US Presidents before and after their terms).

Under times of significant stress, your body wisely prioritizes survival by shifting production from sex hormones (estrogen, progesterone, and testosterone) to stress hormones. This can lead to many hormone imbalance problems such as irregular cycles, PMS, estrogen dominance symptoms, and infertility. In addition, menopause and andropause symptoms nearly always worsen with chronic stress. This was the case with Brenda, whose hormones were balanced for years on her treatment plan, until one day she came in, exasperated, wondering why her symptoms were back:

*Everything's gone completely downhill over the past 2 months. Up until then I was sleeping fine and I had plenty of energy. Now I'm having hot flashes all day long again, and I've gained 10 pounds. I think the pharmacy must have made a mistake in my last prescription.*

When I asked Brenda what was going on in her life, she filled me in:

*I found out recently that my husband's been having an affair. I don't know what I'm going to do about it. I'm also really worried about my son. He dropped out of college and just lays around watching TV all day. I think he might be depressed but he won't see a doctor.*

The pharmacy had not made a mistake in Brenda's prescription. The return of her symptoms was due to her adrenal glands increasing production of stress hormones at the expense of her sex hormones.

Besides contributing to digestive problems, high blood sugar, elevated inflammation, immune dysfunction, fatigue, and other hormone imbalance symptoms, high levels of stress hormones can impact your brain function. When cortisol is released into the bloodstream, the brain responds by increasing output and preventing the reuptake of a neurotransmitter called "glutamate." Prolonged, excessive levels of glutamate are like fire to the brain causing a condition known as "excitotoxicity." Glutamate excess can damage cells in the hippocampus causing short-term memory problems and impaired formation of new memory—such as trouble retrieving words or names, or forgetting things like where you put your keys. Excess cortisol and glutamate also cause a smaller volume, or atrophy, of the hippocampus. With moderate stress this is reversible; however, if stress is severe and prolonged, shrinking of the hippocampus may be permanent.[81]

There is a joke that the word "stressed" is just "desserts" spelled backwards, and many people turn to sweets when they're stressed. This is partly because chronic stress depletes serotonin levels in your brain.[82,83] When serotonin is low you may find yourself eating more refined carbohydrates such as bread, pasta, cookies, and pastries—leading to blood sugar problems, insulin resistance, and weight gain. There is compelling research suggesting that diabetics frequently have low serotonin levels, years before their diagnosis[84]—the low serotonin may fuel their carbohydrate cravings and drive their rising blood sugar. Serotonin deficiency from chronic stress can also contribute to depression and anxiety, migraine headaches, and sleep problems.

My own health history illustrates the relationship between stress and weight gain. When I was in naturopathic medical school, I experienced a great deal of stress—I was overwhelmed with studying, juggling a part-time job, commuting on my bike since I didn't own a car, repeated fasting (because I thought this was healthy), and significant sleep debt from chronic insomnia. During that time I ran marathons and half-marathons, participated in a triathlon, and was very passionate about my exercise and activity level. Although my diet was exceptional, I gained 60 pounds between entering school and finishing my residency. This was the result of significant, prolonged stress and lack of "emptying my stress bucket."

Much of the weight gain related to excess cortisol production is abdominal weight gain, often referred to as belly fat or a "spare tire." Excess weight around the waist means extra fat surrounding abdominal organs, or surplus "visceral fat"—this type of weight gain raises the risk for diabetes, heart disease, and cancer. Chronic stress contributes to weight gain in several different ways:

- Elevated cortisol raises blood sugar, which contributes to insulin resistance.[85,86]

- Abdominal fat cells have up to four times more cortisol receptors than other fat cells.[87]

- The enzyme "11 β-hydroxysteroid dehydrogenase" found in visceral fat cells makes more cortisol from inactive cortisone.[88]

- Cortisol increases appetite.[89]

- Chronic stress depletes serotonin and fuels refined carbohydrate and sugar cravings. [90,91]

- Prolonged, high cortisol levels can decrease thyroid hormone production and function.[92,93]

- Stress stimulates the release of "neuropeptide Y." This neuropeptide induces the formation of new fat cells, and reduces leptin, which strongly increases appetite. [94,95]

You may have noticed your own weight creeping up during times of prolonged stress. It's not important that you understand the mechanism of how stress leads to weight gain—just that you recognize there are many ways that stress promotes weight gain, and that you can do something about it. Chapter 6 will provide tools to lessen the impact stress has on your weight, hormone balance, and longevity.

### Low Thyroid Hormone or Hypothyroidism

Thyroid problems are, unfortunately, the most common endocrine disorder in the U.S. and the prevalence increases with age. Every cell of your body needs thyroid hormone to function properly. This is why low thyroid hormone can lead to symptoms affecting all body systems. As a reminder, thyroid hormone (T4) is made by the thyroid gland after being stimulated by the pituitary via TSH (thyroid stimulating hormone). T4 is then converted into active thyroid hormone, T3. Therefore, hypothyroid symptoms can be due to a pituitary problem, a thyroid gland problem, or a problem converting T4 into active T3. The most common reasons for hypothyroid symptoms are thyroid gland dysfunction and problems converting T4 to active T3. If you're experiencing symptoms of low thyroid hormone, the cause is best determined by blood testing (discussed in chapter 5).

Whatever the reason, low thyroid hormone causes all cells to slow down. This was certainly true for Marilyn, a 72-year-old retired schoolteacher and loving grandmother. Although Marilyn ate a relatively healthy diet and was involved in a walking program with women in her community, she was gaining weight and felt like she couldn't keep up with her schedule anymore. "I feel like I'm walking through molasses," she explained. "I used to be considered an energizer bunny, but I think my battery doesn't hold a charge anymore." Marilyn had gained more than 15 pounds in the past 6 months and noticed changes in her skin and hair, and in her brain:

> My skin is really dry, no matter how much lotion I use. Also, my hair seems dry and brittle, and my hairdresser has commented that it's not growing much. My mind isn't as sharp, either—I have to work hard to figure out what I'm trying to say. And I'm tired and worn down all the time.

Marilyn's lab work revealed she had hypothyroidism because her thyroid gland was unable to make enough hormone. Like Marilyn, most people with hypothyroid symptoms develop fatigue and weakness.

Since the brain needs adequate thyroid hormone, common symptoms of low levels include foggy thinking, mental sluggishness, and forgetfulness. In the US, babies are routinely tested for hypothyroidism at birth to prevent mental retardation.

Thyroid hormone plays a role in regulating the amount of neurotransmitters (brain chemicals) such as serotonin, norepinephrine, and GABA. Active thyroid hormone (T3) has been found in the spaces that connect neurons in the brain.[96] Many people with thyroid hormone deficiency develop depression or anxiety.[97] When a person is hypothyroid, treatment with thyroid hormone can produce dramatic results—when adequately treated, some people comment that their brains work better, "like a light bulb goes on."

People struggling with hypothyroidism often have dry skin and hair, and scalp hair loss. A classic symptom of hypothyroidism is loss of the outer third of the eyebrows and, occasionally, diminished hair growth on the legs.

Water weight gain and puffiness in the face and ankles may occur with hypothyroidism. If the thyroid gland becomes enlarged it can cause trouble swallowing. In addition, some people develop a raspy voice or hoarseness.

Hypothyroidism can cause muscle and joint pain; in fact, it's not uncommon for people with fibromyalgia to have suboptimal thyroid hormone levels. This was certainly the case with Amy, an overworked 32-year-old mother and preschool teacher. Amy had been to her primary care doctor several times over the past year due to her muscle and joint pain and severe fatigue. Amy's doctor sent her to a rheumatologist to make sure she didn't have an autoimmune disease. Since no conventional cause of Amy's pain and fatigue could be found, Amy was told she had fibromyalgia and was counseled to take an antidepressant and over-the-counter pain relievers.

When I measured  Amy's thyroid hormone levels, I was not surprised to see that she had very low active thyroid hormone (T3). Although Amy's thyroid gland was making enough T4, her body was not converting it into active T3. After supplementing with compounded, sustained-release T3 along with selenium and zinc (to enhance the enzyme responsible for converting T4 to T3), and decreasing her stress level, Amy's pain and fatigue significantly improved.

Other symptoms of inadequate thyroid hormone include cold body temperature and reduced sweating from a slow metabolism. When metabolism slows, the body conserves calories leading to weight gain. Decreased digestion from hypothyroidism can lead to constipation. In addition, thyroid deficiency may cause elevated LDL (bad) cholesterol and blockages in the arteries. Eventually, long-term, untreated hypothyroidism can lead to coronary artery disease, enlargement of the heart, and congestive heart failure.

The following symptoms and conditions may be due to low thyroid hormone:

- fatigue
- weight gain
- muscle pain
- intolerance to cold
- depression
- forgetfulness
- enlarged thyroid (goiter)
- dry skin or hair

- hair loss
- hoarse voice
- constipation
- heart disease
- congestive heart failure
- high cholesterol
- infertility and miscarriage

## Hormone Imbalance and Weight Gain

You've likely heard these alarming statistics: one-third of children in the US are overweight and 17% are clinically obese. Two thirds of adults are considered overweight, and 33% are obese. By 2015 it is estimated that 75% of Americans will be overweight or obese.

Being overweight increases the risk of heart disease, type 2 diabetes, breast cancer, high blood pressure, gallstones, osteoarthritis, and sleep apnea. In fact, the International Agency for Research on Cancer (part of the World Health Organization) attributes 25-33% of cancers of the breast, colon, uterus, esophagus, and kidney, to physical inactivity and being overweight. Nearly all health experts agree — obesity is a national health crisis.

Hormone imbalance certainly contributes to the epidemic of overweight and obesity. The most significant hormone imbalance involved in weight gain is too much insulin production. Excess insulin can disrupt all other hormones and cause a whirlwind of damage. Recall that insulin is made in response to blood sugar, so chronically elevated blood sugar causes excessive insulin production. Insulin is your fat storage hormone — the higher your insulin level, the more fat tissue you will store. Elevated insulin levels also accelerate aging and contribute to chronic inflammation and degenerative disease.

As you learned in the section on adrenal excess and fatigue, prolonged stress and high cortisol levels can lead to weight gain through several mechanisms. These include contributing to insulin resistance, increasing appetite, lowering thyroid hormone function, and even decreasing testosterone production. As you now know, testosterone is the hormone that promotes muscle mass and strength and improves lean body mass (muscle to fat ratio). Therefore, suboptimal testosterone can contribute to weight problems in both men and women. Low testosterone and high estrogen (especially in men) can also exacerbate insulin resistance.

Achieving and maintaining hormone balance between insulin, cortisol, thyroid hormone, testosterone, and estrogen is crucial in keeping your body lean and fit.

# Chapter 5: Testing

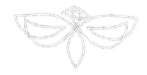

You now know that hormone levels decline with age. This is known as menopause in women, andropause in men, and adrenopause (declining DHEA) in women and men. Hypothyroidism is also more common with aging. You also know that, when hormones decline, aging accelerates.

So what can you do about it?

First, become educated about what hormones do and what symptoms of hormone imbalance you may have. After reading the previous chapters, you may have some idea if you suffer from hormone imbalance. Lab testing can verify hormone levels and provide a blueprint for treatment.

In addition to hormone testing, there are other optimal aging tests that can clarify the picture of your current health. These include DNA testing to identify your genetic susceptibility for certain diseases and health conditions; oxidative stress, antioxidant, and Coenzyme Q10 levels to determine free radical status and antioxidant need; and testing telomere length to assess the biological age of your cells. These advanced laboratory tests can enable you and your physician to create a unique, individualized treatment plan based on your current health and genetic susceptibilities.

## Normal isn't Optimal

When performing hormone testing, it's important to note that the interpretation of your results matters. Often times laboratories report "normal" ranges that may not be optimal. This is true for "normal" ranges of all of the sex hormones (estradiol, progesterone, and testosterone), as well as DHEA and thyroid hormone.

An example where interpretation matters is assessing optimal testosterone levels. Testosterone is often reported by laboratories in terms of average levels for a given age in men. Although declining testosterone is common (which often gets called "normal") it isn't necessarily optimal. Arguably, testosterone levels in the upper range for men aged 21 to 40, when men are at their physical peak, could be considered optimal for men. In addition, low testosterone levels in women—even lower than the detection limit of the test—are often reported as "within the normal range." Clearly the word "normal" in this case does not mean optimal.

Another example where interpretation matters is in assessing ideal thyroid levels. Physicians usually rely on the TSH (thyroid stimulating hormone) test to evaluate the overall amount of hormone produced by the thyroid gland. TSH is made by your pituitary—its function is to stimulate the thyroid gland to make thyroid hormone. When thyroid output is low, TSH increases. Reference ranges are determined by measuring supposedly healthy people in the general population. Currently, many laboratories report a "normal" TSH as 0.5 to 5.5 µIU/mL, and doctors diagnose hypothyroidism if a TSH level is >5.5. However, many individuals with TSH levels in the upper end of the reference range may actually be suffering from hypothyroid symptoms and conditions (such as elevated cholesterol, heart disease, infertility, and depression). This has led the American Association of Clinical Endocrinologists (AACE) in 2003 to develop a narrower TSH reference range of 0.3 to 3.0 µIU/mL, with the hope that "the new range will result in improved accuracy of diagnosis for millions of Americans who suffer from a mild thyroid disorder, but who have gone untreated."[98] Other endocrine organizations such as The Endocrine Society and the American Thyroid Association are in agreement with the AACE position. Unfortunately, many doctors are unfamiliar with this recommendation and mistakenly tell patients with TSH levels >3.0 and hypothyroid symptoms or conditions that they don't need treatment.

As you can see, embracing an "optimal vs. normal" mindset is important when interpreting lab results. The Life Extension Foundation and ZRT Laboratory have worked to establish optimal reference ranges for hormone testing (see chapter 9 for more information). Many physicians specializing in anti-aging medicine today understand the importance of optimal levels when reviewing lab results.

## Necessary Hormone and Blood Tests for Women

If you're a woman who is still having periods, it's important to test hormones when you're not menstruating (estradiol and progesterone are very low during menses). Testosterone levels are relatively stable throughout the cycle, although testosterone does peak right before ovulation (in the middle of the cycle). Progesterone increases after ovulation (usually mid-cycle) and peaks between days 19 and 21 in a regular, 28-day cycle. FSH (follicle stimulating hormone), made by the pituitary, helps determine how happy the brain is with overall estrogen production. When FSH is >23 mIU/ml, it indicates low estrogen levels and likely peri or postmenopausal status. Often times the higher the FSH, the worse the estrogen-deficiency symptoms. It is also necessary to test levels of estradiol, progesterone, and total and free testosterone.

Since DHEA is the precursor for production of the sex hormones, and is needed for healthy brain and immune function, it's helpful to test DHEA-S, or "DHEA-sulphate" (DHEA levels fluctuate—DHEA-S is a better indicator of overall DHEA production).

Screening for low thyroid function can be performed by measuring a TSH level; testing free T4 and free T3 can add information about thyroid hormone production and conversion to active thyroid hormone.

Testing vitamin D levels for bone and cancer prevention is important. In addition, a fasting blood glucose level can help determine the possibility of diabetes or insulin resistance, as can a hemoglobin A1C (which determines blood sugar levels for the previous three months). Essential blood tests for pre and postmenopausal women include:

- FSH
- Estradiol
- Progesterone
- Total and free testosterone
- DHEA-S, or DHEA-sulphate
- TSH, free T4, free T3
- Fasting glucose & hemoglobin A1C

- 25-OH vitamin D (most accurate measurement of total body vitamin D)

## *Optional Tests for Women*

If a woman is experiencing heavy menses or significant fatigue, it is important to screen for anemia. In addition, determining cortisol levels can help establish health of the adrenal glands and enhance the picture of hormone imbalance. Note: cortisol testing is best performed by saliva testing; salivary cortisol testing has been shown to be highly accurate.[99-102] Optional tests for women include:

- CBC (complete blood count) — to rule out anemia or white blood cell problem
- Cortisol (via saliva testing)
- Lipid panel — to determine triglyceride and cholesterol levels. Poor lipid profiles may be due to hormone imbalance (e.g., insulin resistance, low testosterone, or low thyroid hormone)
- High sensitivity or cardio C-reactive protein — helps evaluate cardiovascular risk

## *Necessary Hormone and Blood Tests for Men*

Men should receive tests to determine total and free testosterone levels, PSA to screen for prostate cancer, and estradiol levels to make sure they aren't converting too much testosterone into estrogen. Since testosterone levels are highest in the morning (especially in younger men), it's best to have your blood drawn before 9:00 am. In addition, testing hemoglobin and hematocrit levels is necessary to look for anemia, or for hemochromatosis or polycythemia vera (conditions in which testosterone supplementation would be contraindicated).

Fasting glucose and hemoglobin A1C levels will reveal the likelihood of diabetes or insulin resistance, and 25-OH vitamin D can evaluate bone health and cancer risk. Although hypothyroidism is less common in men than in women, it is important to test TSH levels in men, and possibly free T4 and free T3 levels. Lastly, measuring DHEA-sulphate, which indicates overall DHEA production, can provide more information to maintain brain and immune system health. Necessary tests include:

- Total & free testosterone

- Estradiol
- PSA
- TSH, free T4, free T3
- DHEA-S
- Fasting glucose & hemoglobin A1C
- 25-OH vitamin D
- Hemoglobin & hematocrit
- Chemistry screen including liver and kidney function tests

## Optional Tests for Men

- LH (luteinizing hormone) & FSH (follicle stimulating hormone) — these pituitary hormones help differentiate between aging, pituitary, or other causes of low testosterone. This test may not be as important in men over 50.
- Cortisol (via saliva testing)
- Lipid panel — to determine triglyceride and cholesterol levels. Poor lipid profiles may be due to hormone imbalance (e.g., insulin resistance, low testosterone, or low thyroid hormone)
- High sensitivity or cardio C-reactive protein — helps evaluate cardiovascular risk

## Other Testing: Genetic Susceptibility

The recent availability of inexpensive genetic susceptibility testing is a remarkable medical achievement. This testing determines single nucleotide polymorphisms or SNPs (pronounced "snips"), which are changes in DNA that can predispose you to certain diseases and health problems.

Remember, even if you test positive for certain SNPs, you still retain the power to change your health destiny — because you can control how your genes are expressed. If you undertake SNP testing, it is crucial that you understand this: your SNPs may increase your risk for certain diseases, but the choices you make every day — what you eat, whether or not you exercise, how you live, what environment you surround yourself with, and which supplements you take — will determine most of your health destiny.

SNP testing is available to determine risk for the following conditions:

- Detoxification capacity and drug metabolism
- Osteoporosis
- Cardiovascular disease
- Nutrient or supplementation needs
- B6 metabolism — to assess whether or not you need higher dosages or bioavailable forms, such as pyridoxyl-5-phosphate
- Folate metabolism — to determine the ability to make active folic acid (called MTHF, or methyl-tetrahydrofolate)
- Brain health and risk for neurodegenerative disorders
- Mood disorders such as anxiety and depression
- Oxidative stress
- Immune function and risk for infections, allergies, autoimmune diseases, and certain cancers
- Increased tendency to produce inflammation

### Free Radicals, Antioxidant Status, and Coenzyme Q10

Besides testing your hormones and genetic susceptibility, you can choose to test your free radical and antioxidant levels. When testing free radical levels, you are discovering your body's level of oxidative stress. Oxidative stress occurs when the production of reactive oxygen species (oxygen ions, free radicals, and peroxides) outweighs your body's ability to remove them.

When free radical production exceeds removal, it tips the balance in the direction of oxidation — or rusting. These free radicals steal electrons from nearby molecules in ways that cause a chain reaction, ultimately damaging cells, proteins, and DNA.

Oxidative stress has been implicated in a growing list of disorders including cancer, atherosclerosis, arthritis, diabetes, macular degeneration, chronic fatigue syndrome, fibromyalgia, neurodegenerative diseases (such as dementia, Alzheimer's, and Parkinson's), and of course, aging itself.

Antioxidants extinguish free radicals and render them harmless. Different people will need different amounts and types of antioxidants. Blood antioxidant testing is available to measure your levels of vitamin E (alpha & gamma tocopherol), vitamin C, vitamin A, beta-carotene, lutein, lycopene, and coenzyme Q10.

## Telomere Testing

This last type of "optimal aging" testing is quite new and exciting. Telomere testing has been available in the research setting for several years. Recently, however, this testing is available for you to determine your biological age—the actual age of your cells. Recall from chapter one that telomeres are sections of DNA at the end of chromosomes, similar to the protective plastic caps ("aglets") on the ends of a shoelace. Telomeres shorten every time a cell replicates; when they shorten below a certain threshold, DNA starts to become damaged during replication, conditions associated with aging appear, and cells die. Telomere length is affected by age, genetics, lifestyle, disease, and certain drugs. Telomeres are shortened by oxidative stress and antioxidant deficiencies, as well as by a sedentary lifestyle, nutrient deficiencies, stress, and excess weight.

For more information about testing, please see the "Resources" list in chapter 9.

# Chapter 6: Natural ways to regain and maintain hormone balance

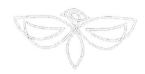

## *Causes of Hormone Imbalance*

You now know that hormone imbalance is common with aging, and that aging accelerates when hormone levels decline. You also know that lab testing is available to determine your hormone levels, inherited genetic susceptibilities (SNPs), biological age of your cells (telomere testing), and to assess antioxidant needs. Lab work can provide a map to guide your plan for slowing or reversing the effects of aging.

Your plan also requires an understanding of the four major causes of hormone imbalance—stress, poor diet & lifestyle habits, toxicity, and aging. You'll notice that the only cause of hormone imbalance you cannot control is chronological aging.

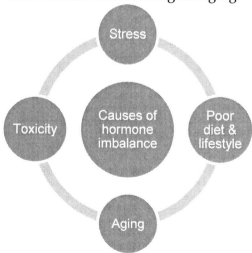

Recognizing the causes of hormone imbalance that are within your control—stress, poor diet & lifestyle habits, and toxicity—will empower you to make necessary changes and health-affirming choices to achieve HormoneSynergy and optimal aging. The foundations for treatment are referred to as **The 8 Steps for Achieving HormoneSynergy.** Although these eight steps could become a book themselves, they're summarized here with the hope that you'll implement some or all of them into your life right now.

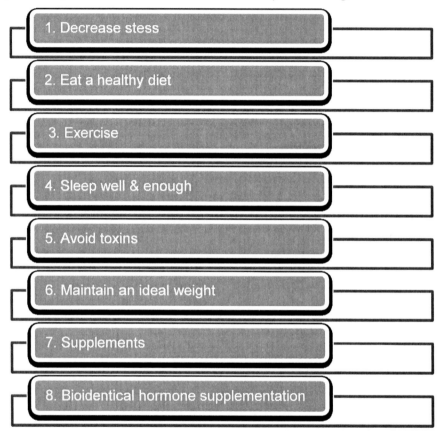

## *The 8 Steps for Achieving HormoneSynergy:*

- Decrease stress
- Eat a healthy diet & keep your blood sugar balanced
- Exercise
- Sleep well & enough
- Avoid toxins and do a yearly detox

- Maintain an ideal weight, including muscle and fat percentages
- Supplements: multi-vitamins & minerals, antioxidants including CoQ10, vitamin D, resveratrol, and fish oil
- Bioidentical hormone supplementation, weighing your individual risks and benefits

The rest of this chapter summarizes the first seven steps, and offers tools to enable you to perform them on a daily basis. These seven steps are fundamental in achieving optimal aging. The eighth step — bioidentical hormone supplementation — is the subject of chapter eight.

### Step 1: Decrease stress.

You may recall from chapter four that the feelings and symptoms of stress are due to a sequence of biochemical events in your body. Technically, stress is not an actual event or circumstance — it's your body's reaction to an event or circumstance. This means that stress is not <u>what</u> happens to you — it's <u>how you respond</u> to what happens to you. You have the ability to control how you respond to events and circumstances in your life and to diminish the impact stress has on your body.

It's essential to remember that your body responds to stress, whether it's real — such as being chased by a swarm of bees — or perceived — such as feeling trapped in a traffic jam — the same way. And your body benefits tremendously from releasing stress or "emptying your stress bucket" every day.

Many things can trigger a stress response. Psychological stressors you may experience include worry, time pressure, or unresolved emotions. Sometimes environmental factors can trigger a stress response — for example, too much noise, or excess nighttime stimulation of your brain from staying up late on the computer or watching a disturbing TV show. Pain, infection, surgery, over-exercising, and poor sleep will also trigger a stress response. Lastly, dieting and food deprivation will be interpreted by your body as a threat, and when the body is threatened, it sounds the alarm.

Now that you understand how repeated or prolonged stress can damage your body and cause rapid aging, you likely recognize how crucial it is to lower stress on a daily basis. Start practicing the following strategies — stop creating emergencies, avoid being a victim, slow down, do one thing at a time, and laugh and have fun — to empty your stress bucket every day.

## Stop Creating Emergencies

Recognizing what situations trigger a stress response and avoiding them is crucial. One way to decrease the number of times a day you trigger your own stress response is to differentiate between emergencies and non-emergencies. The stress response was designed to save your life in true emergencies, not for situations that you may treat as emergencies even though they're not.

Several years ago, my dog Libby taught me this valuable lesson. One afternoon, my husband, Libby, and I were walking on a path near our home. Another dog approached, pulling ahead of its owner on the leash. When the two dogs crossed paths, the other dog jumped on Libby and they became a snarling, barking pair. We pulled them apart and continued our walk — Libby immediately went back to sniffing trees and trotting along in the grass. If Libby had been a human, she would likely have responded much differently — perhaps exclaiming how unfair it was that she was attacked unprovoked, or that the other dog's owner should have had better control over her dog. As we continued our walk I never heard Libby worry about future dogs she might encounter, nor did I hear her rehash the incident with the dog that jumped on her. In fact, to this day, Libby has never re-lived (and recreated the stress of) that incident! Humans would certainly lower their stress if we followed Libby's example — *wag more, bark less.*

The lesson Libby taught me is that of the difference between animals and humans — animals respond to stress when provoked, that is, the stress and the response are in the present moment. Humans create chronic stress through anticipation (worry) and rehashing past situations. Please remember this: *your body increases cortisol production from imagined threats just as it does from real ones. When you stop creating emergencies, you will lower your stress level.*

This is not to imply that discussing past trauma isn't valuable — acknowledging the past can enable you to heal deep wounds and prevent future pain. For your health's sake, emphasis should be placed on releasing the past and learning how to prevent triggering stress responses when they're not necessary. If you recognize a pattern of creating emergencies, work with a therapist or certified Life Coach to help you respond differently in the future. In addition, Eckhart Tolle's books *The Power of Now* and *Stillness Speaks* are excellent tools for learning to be in the present moment. Chapter 9 offers additional resources.

## Avoid Being a Victim

Nobody is responsible for your stress. Not your parents, spouse, boss, or kids; not the economy, God, anyone, or anything else. Although this has already been stated, it's worth repeating: stress is not <u>what</u> happens to you, it's <u>how you respond</u> to what happens to you. You have control over how you respond to things that happen in your life. When you truly grasp this concept, your life will change.

If you find yourself in a situation that repeatedly causes you stress, it may be helpful to remember your options (there are four):

1. Work to change the situation. Acknowledge what you can and cannot do, and work on what you can change.

2. Accept the situation. You may have already worked on what you can change about the situation. Accepting the way things are is not the same as giving up. It simply means you drop your resistance and reaction to the situation—no resistance or reaction, no stress.

3. Leave or remove yourself from the situation. If the situation that's provoking your stress is unacceptable and unchangeable, leaving may be the best or only way to preserve your health.

4. Do none of the above. If the situation is unacceptable, you're not able or willing to work to change it (or your response to it), and you stay in the situation, recognize that this is a decision that will affect your health. If you find yourself stuck in a stress-inducing situation, keep re-evaluating the above steps—eventually, you may be able to respond in a more health-affirming way.

## Slow Down

The Greek philosopher Heraclitus once said, "A man cannot step in the same river twice," meaning that humans are constantly changing, as are rivers and everything else in the world. Now that you know how stress can significantly damage your health, you will likely be more aware of the times you create avoidable stress in your life. The next time you find yourself rushing somewhere, become aware of this, and slow down. You only need to slow down a fraction of a second to become mindful of the present moment, and to turn off the stress response.

If hurrying is a pattern for you, consider attaching a note saying *"Slow down"* or *"Be here, now"* to the dashboard of your car or refrigerator, or leave yourself a reminder on your computer or cell phone monitor—this will serve as an anchor to the present moment.

## Do One Thing at a Time

In today's world, we're often bombarded with phone calls, emails, text messages, and other interruptions while performing everyday tasks. You may think that multitasking saves time and enables you to be more efficient, however, some studies have exposed this as a myth. In one study, researchers from the Federal Aviation Administration and the University of Michigan teamed up to perform experiments where participants alternated between different tasks ("multitasked") or performed the same task repeatedly. The researchers found that participants lost time with multitasking, and the time lost increased with complexity of the tasks.[103] What this means is that multitasking may seem more efficient on the surface, but it can actually cost you time in the end.

In another study by a group of Stanford University researchers, people who identified as regular multitaskers were actually worse at ignoring extraneous stimuli than people who preferred to do one thing at a time. Not only were the regular multitaskers more distractible, they weren't any better at switching between different tasks. In addition, they made more mistakes in remembering information presented while multitasking.[104]

It seems impossible to avoid all multitasking in today's world. Avoiding it when you can, however, may help prevent your stress bucket from overflowing. Consider scheduling "email checking" times, rather than incessantly looking at your computer, Blackberry, or iPhone inbox. Also, commit to only driving while driving—in other words, don't combine driving with other activities such as eating, talking on your cell phone, or putting on mascara. Consider adopting the personal habit of financial adviser, Suze Orman—an advocate of doing one thing at a time. In an interview with *Time*, she says she has strict rules on using electronic devices. For example, she has a cell phone but doesn't leave it on, reasoning, "You have to stop thinking you are at everyone's beck and call. You cannot complete your thoughts with everything ringing."[105]

## Laugh and Have Fun Every Day

Patients often find it funny when I write them a prescription that says, "Do something fun every day" with an unlimited number of refills! As adults, we often forget that life is not all about work and responsibilities. Prioritizing playtime for yourself can be key in emptying your stress bucket since fun and laugher have been shown to improve health and lower cortisol levels.[106-108] Of course, what's fun for someone else may not be fun for you, so figure out what activities make you smile, laugh, or feel joyful, and do one or many of them every day—doctor's orders!

If you're stuck on what to do to meet your "laugh and play daily" prescription, consider the leisure activities evaluated in one aspect of the Einstein Study published in the New England Journal of Medicine. In this study, researchers looked at many different thinking and physical activities and the risk for dementia. The results showed that reading, participating in board games, playing musical instruments, and dancing were most effective at preventing cognitive decline.[109] The more frequent your participation in leisure activities, the sharper your mind may remain.

Not only do laughing and having fun lower cortisol and keep your brain sharp, they also improve your immune system by enhancing natural killer cell function (the cells that destroy cancer cells) and promoting secretory IgA production.[110,111] Secretory IgA plays a critical role in the immune system of mucus membranes in the gastrointestinal and respiratory systems, and the health of the vagina and prostate. This means that having fun may prevent cancer, and may inhibit microbes from causing infections in your respiratory, gastrointestinal, and reproductive systems.

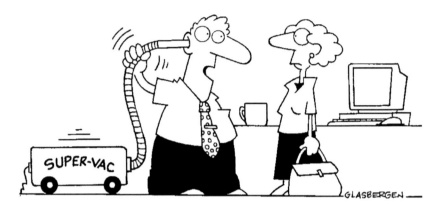

"It's just something I do every day at 5:00
to get rid of stress before I go home."

### Step 2: Eat a healthy diet and keep your blood sugar balanced.

Hippocrates is credited with saying, "Let your food be your medicine, and your medicine be your food." Besides a healthy diet being "good medicine," food is literally what your body uses to build tissue and perform daily functions—in other words, <u>you literally become what you eat</u>.

Remember back in chapter one when you learned that your genes make up your "book of life"? Keep in mind that your genes are not your destiny—it's the way your genes express themselves (or how your book of life is "read") that determines who you are. Food is a critical part of this process—food provides the signaling substances that tell your genes what to do. In other words, <u>food is information for your genes.</u> The next time you eat something, ask yourself, *"Am I feeding my genes good information?"* If the answer is "yes," you are providing your body with a powerful substance that influences your rate of aging and risk for disease.

### The purpose of food

All food can be categorized into three main groups—protein, fat, and carbohydrates.

Protein is used for tissue and cell structures, to make hormones and neurotransmitters (brain chemicals), and for antibody production for your immune system. Therefore, high quality, adequate protein is critical to build healthy bones, muscles, skin, and organs; it's also necessary for ideal hormone balance, brain health, and immune function. Good quality protein sources include vegetarian options such as whey, soy, beans, and nuts. Animal products such as dairy, eggs, lean meat, and fish are also good protein sources. To limit your exposure to toxins, it's best to eat free-range meat and wild caught fish, and to avoid fish high in heavy metals such as tuna and swordfish.

Fats play a role in hormone balance since they are used to make some hormones. For example, cholesterol is the backbone for estrogen, progesterone, testosterone, DHEA, cortisol, and vitamin D synthesis. This is why reducing your cholesterol too much can lead to hormone deficiencies. Fats also make up your cell walls as well as receptors that serve as hormone binding sites. The brain is made up of 60% fat, approximately 25% of which is omega three fatty acids (such as those found in fish oil). In addition, fat is necessary to absorb vitamins A, D, E, K, and carotenoids. Fat also provides a source for energy production and a place to store it.

Nearly all food contains some amount of fat. The total amount of fat you eat isn't nearly as important as the type of fat. "Good fats," including monounsaturated and polyunsaturated fatty acids, help lower disease risk. Monounsaturated fats are found in olive oil, as well as nuts such as almonds, pecans, cashews, and hazelnuts. Good sources of polyunsaturated fats include flaxseed, grapeseed, and fish oils. Omega-3 fatty acids are a type of polyunsaturated fatty acid.

"Bad" fats include too much saturated fat and all trans fats. Saturated fat is necessary for health; however, your body can create it so it isn't an essential fat, and most people eat too much of it. Trans fats are made by heating liquid vegetable oils in the presence of hydrogen (hence the name, "hydrogenated oil"). Trans fats are used in the processed food industry because they're more stable and less likely to oxidize or spoil. Trans fats are known to damage arteries and the heart and to increase inflammation. Trans fats also contribute to obesity, insulin resistance, and diabetes. The average American eats six grams of trans fat per day (ideally this should be zero). Besides increasing the risk for heart attacks and strokes, trans fats increase breast cancer risk.[112] It's relatively easy to avoid eating any trans fats—stay away from commercially packaged baked goods, snack foods, and fast food. Don't eat any food with "partially hydrogenated oil" on the label, avoid margarine and shortening, and don't eat fried food in restaurants.

The last food category, carbohydrates, provides your cells with their main source of fuel. The best sources of carbohydrates—vegetables, fruits, beans, and whole grains—contain fiber, vitamins, and minerals. Fruits and vegetables are great sources of phytonutrients, including antioxidants. To prevent internal "rusting" and keep free radicals to a minimum, make sure you eat at least 5-7 servings of vegetables and fruit every day.

Since insulin rises in response to increasing blood sugar levels, it's important to avoid carbohydrates that cause rapid spikes in blood sugar. Remember that high insulin disrupts all other hormones and body systems; it also causes weight gain, accelerates aging, and leads to chronic inflammation and degenerative disease.

To determine the effect different carbohydrate-rich foods have on your blood sugar, consult the glycemic index. The glycemic index is a ranking of carbohydrates from 0 to 100 according to the amount they raise blood sugar. Foods with a high glycemic index (e.g., white bread, potatoes, rice milk) are quickly digested and absorbed, rapidly increasing blood sugar. Foods low on the glycemic-index are digested and absorbed more slowly and cause a gradual and sustained rise in blood sugar and insulin levels. The "International Glycemic Index Database," maintained by the University of Sydney in Australia, is available at www.glycemicindex.com. You may also consider the foods you eat in terms of their glycemic load. The glycemic load is similar to the glycemic index except it takes into account the quantity of carbohydrate commonly eaten for specific foods.

With all the hype about the health benefits of alcohol, many people believe alcohol is the new health food. Red wine is, indeed, an excellent source of antioxidants (so are the grapes it's made from) as well as resveratrol (more on this in "Step 7: Supplements"). Alcohol has been shown to reduce the risk of heart attack and stroke, and may decrease the risk for developing type 2 diabetes.[113,114] Unfortunately, many people overindulge without regard for the negative health consequences of alcohol, or the excess, "empty" calories it contains. Moderate alcohol intake is defined as no more than two drinks for men, and one drink for women, per day. Studies have shown that high alcohol intake increases aromatization of androgens to estrogen, and impedes the liver's ability to clear excess estrogen from the body. In women, more than one drink per day can increase breast cancer risk. In men, more than two drinks per day boost estrogen levels within the liver[115] and may lead to weight gain in the waist and the development of "man boobs." Heavy drinking in men—defined as four or more drinks per day, five or more days per week—increases the risk for aggressive forms of prostate cancer.[116]

When designing your ideal diet, think about the information you want to provide your genes with, and focus on what you should eat every day. This is more effective than focusing on what you shouldn't eat, and fighting with yourself to avoid fueling your genes with garbage. Ask yourself daily if you've met your body's nutritional needs: 5-7 servings of vegetables and fruit, good quality protein, healthy fats, and whole grains. Think about how you'll incorporate your 5-7 servings of vegetables and fruit in your daily meals and make sure you plan ahead—remember the adage, "*If you fail to plan, you plan to fail*".

It's also helpful to treat your body like an unrepeatable, sacred place (because it is)—you wouldn't dump garbage into a temple, mosque, or church so please don't do this to your body.

Remember to start your day with a breakfast high in protein (eggs, lean meat, yogurt, protein powders) and low-glycemic index carbohydrates. In addition, eat protein three times a day to prevent "roller coaster" blood sugar levels and sugar cravings throughout the day. If you do indulge in alcohol, be honest with yourself about the amount and frequency.

Now that you know how crucial the food you eat is to your health, prevention of chronic disease, and aging, be mindful of the quality of food you choose (and the information you provide your genes with) every meal, every day.

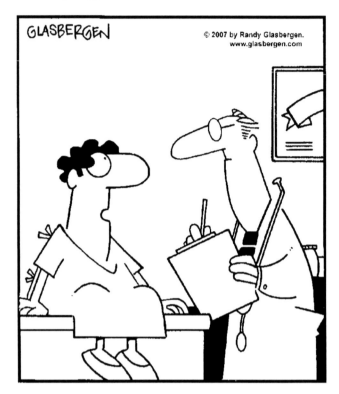

**"Don't tell me to improve my diet. I ate
a carrot once and nothing happened!"**

### Step 3: Exercise.

The percentage of Americans who do not exercise is alarming: 40% of the population is completely sedentary, and fewer than 20% get enough exercise for cardiovascular benefit.

Remember Newton's first law? A body at rest, stays at rest. Newton's law is the reason it's necessary to keep your body moving by incorporating exercise into your life every day. In other words, a body in motion stays in motion! Since exercise raises growth hormone, think of it as the most important anti-aging remedy you take—and it must be performed for 30-45 minutes, every 24 to 48 hours.

Although the benefits of exercise seem obvious, it may be helpful to highlight a few. First, exercise lowers estrogen in men (less fat, less aromatase) and raises testosterone in women and men, as long as the exercise isn't excessive.[117,118] Testosterone elevation is seen after about 20 minutes of exercise, and lasts for one to three hours. In addition, exercise strengthens bone and muscle, including the heart muscle. Exercise is also one of the most effective ways to promote insulin sensitivity and reverse insulin resistance. Research has shown that exercise lowers your risk for heart disease, diabetes, dementia, depression, and cancer.

If improving health and mood, decreasing the risk for chronic diseases, and promoting longevity isn't enough of a motivator for you to exercise, you may be swayed by the fact that people who exercise have been shown to have more active sex lives and better orgasms.[119] Sometimes knowledge is a powerful motivator!

If you're a member of the 40% of Americans who are completely sedentary, commit to quitting that club right now and start where you are in terms of increasing activity. Your goal may be to merely get off the couch and walk for one minute, turn around and walk home. The next day, you may walk 2 minutes, and so on. If you're ready to exercise at the intensity and frequency needed to significantly benefit your heart, brain, and body, please heed the following advice:

- If you have any heart problems, chest pain, shortness of breath, or injuries, check with your doctor before beginning an exercise plan.
- Choose activities you enjoy and vary them (cross-train).
- Set realistic goals including frequency, intensity, and time (F.I.T.).

F = frequency (days/week)

I = intensity or % maximum heart rate

T = time per session (or each day)

To achieve ideal weight and cardiovascular benefit, you must exercise at the intensity where your heart rate is 60 to 80% of its maximum. To determine your target heart rate, fill in these blanks:

Maximum heart rate = 220 – age: _____

Multiply by 0.6 = _____

Multiply by 0.8 = _____

My target heart rate = _____ to _____ beats per minute.

Yoda's famous words *"Do or do no – there is no try"* remind us that commitment is the first step to achieving a goal. If you are not exercising enough, make the following commitment <u>aloud</u>, right now. You may want to declare this commitment to someone who loves you, as a way of cementing your promise to yourself and others.

*I believe that exercise is extremely important for my brain and body's health.*

*I commit to making exercise a priority in my life.*

*I will find one or more reasons to stay motivated.*

Consider repeating this mantra throughout the day as a way to train your subconscious mind to support your exercise promise. If you find yourself reneging on your commitment, it may be helpful to listen to hypnosis or guided visualization CDs, or enlist the expertise of a personal trainer or Certified Life Coach. See resources in chapter 9 for more ideas.

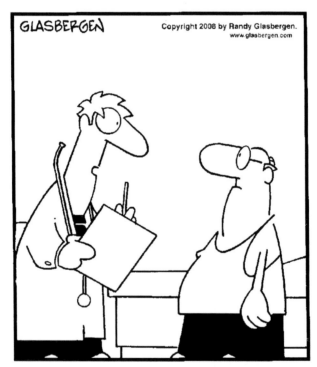

**"What fits your busy schedule better,
exercising one hour a day or being
dead 24 hours a day?"**

## Step 4: Sleep well and enough.

I often tell my patients there are two panaceas in medicine: sleep and exercise. This means that sleep and exercise support your vital force — your inherent ability to heal and maintain wellness — no matter what your health problems. This is in part because both sleep and exercise raise growth hormone production in your body. Remember that growth hormone is responsible for repair of your body's tissues — when growth hormone levels decline, aging rapidly accelerates.

Sleep is also important because melatonin levels are highest during sleep and darkness. Lower melatonin production, seen in people who work the "graveyard" shift, is associated with an increased risk of colon, breast, and prostate cancers.[120-124] In fact, the International Agency for Research on Cancer, part of the World Health Organization, has stated that graveyard shift working and its disruption of the circadian rhythm is a probable carcinogen.[125] Melatonin is a very potent antioxidant with the ability to suppress the growth of cancerous tumors.[126,127]

Although sleep researchers still don't completely understand all the reasons we sleep and dream, your body performs several known activities during sleep. One of the most important functions of sleep is memory consolidation. If you're having trouble with your memory, especially regarding things you've just learned, make sure you're getting enough sleep. In addition, your brain processes the events of your day during sleep. Lastly, sleep allows time for your body to repair damage caused by daily metabolism, stress, ultraviolet radiation, and toxic exposure.

Although most people have trouble sleeping from time to time, chronic sleep deprivation has been linked to health problems such as depression and decreased concentration. Moreover, lack of sleep can weaken your immune system and prevent wounds from healing. Certain medical conditions are more common with inadequate sleep including heart disease, high blood pressure, and diabetes.[128,129] Inadequate sleep raises a hormone called "ghrelin," which stimulates appetite and can lead to being overweight or obese.[130,131]

How much sleep are you getting? Do you wake rested and rejuvenated? If not, you likely didn't sleep long or well enough. Ideally, you should sleep for 7-9 hours a night. If you're not sleeping well or enough, recognize this as a health problem and commit to doing something about it. If you snore or your bed partner says you stop breathing at times, see a sleep medicine specialist. If you're struggling with sleep problems, follow these guidelines:

- Be consistent with your bedtime and awakening time as much as possible. Allow yourself a chance to unwind before hitting the pillow and plan for at least 15 to 30 minutes to fall asleep. Your body gets used to falling asleep at a certain time if you keep your bedtime consistent.

- Make sure your bed is comfortable. Since you spend approximately one-third of your life sleeping, invest in a bed that suits your body.

- Keep your room cool, especially if you're hot at night or have night sweats. Your body temperature decreases as you fall asleep, therefore, taking a hot bath and sleeping in a cool environment can enhance this effect. Keep your bedroom between 55 and 75 degrees.

- Maintain darkness since light suppresses melatonin, your sleep hormone. Even small amounts of light, such as a clock radio or streetlight shining through the window, can be enough to keep you up. If you use the bathroom in the middle of the night, try doing so in the dark or keep a small penlight next to the bed to light your way.

- Ditch the TV and computer from your bedroom. Both provide excitatory stimuli to the brain at a time when you're trying to induce a calming state. In addition, news or disturbing TV shows can occupy your thoughts, preventing you from having sweet dreams.

- If you're in pain, use adequate pain management. Many people are concerned about getting "hooked" on pain medication, even though their pain keeps them up at night. If you are in pain and it keeps you from sleeping, remember inadequate sleep can prevent healing, increase inflammation, and worsen your pain. There are many different ways to treat pain, long and short-term, and you are not "weak," nor is it a sign of failure, to need pain medication in order to sleep. Make sure your doctor knows if pain keeps you from sleeping, and ask for a referral to a pain specialist if you need it.

- Avoid alcohol before bed. Although alcohol may help you fall asleep, you may find yourself awake a few hours later. This is because your brain becomes stimulated as the alcohol is metabolized and cleared from your blood stream.

- Stop all caffeine after noon. The half-life of caffeine increases with aging; therefore, it can remain in your system longer (up to 14 hours)  and you may awaken more often during the night.

- Don't eat a heavy meal before bed and stop fluid intake after 8:00 pm. You may experience reflux or digestive problems if you lie down with a full stomach, and not drinking in the evening may help prevent waking from the need to urinate.

- Exercise daily! (However, not within two hours of bedtime). Exercise has consistently been shown to promote healthy sleep. A word of caution: please do not sacrifice sleep for exercise. If you must choose due to time constraints, exercise for less time and sleep more. Then, re-evaluate your schedule to prioritize sleep and exercise over other time-consumers that aren't promoting your health (such as TV or surfing the Internet.)

- Begin a "worry" and "gratitude" journal. Write down your worries or concerns before going to sleep. Tell yourself that you will attend to your worries the next day, but that your intention is to repair your body and brain by sleeping for the next several hours. Consider writing from a chair or room other than your bedroom so you avoid anchoring your bed to your worries. Finish your "worry list" with at least five things for which you are grateful. Assigning a "worry time" can help you compartmentalize concerns so you don't spend sleep time ruminating (and creating stress hormones). In addition, keeping the things you're grateful for in your awareness will help you fall asleep with positive thoughts.

- Listen to a guided visualization or self-hypnosis CD before bed or if you wake up. These tools support your subconscious mind in allowing you to sleep. Self-hypnosis is completely safe (you will not do things out of your control while listening to a hypnosis CD). See the Resources section in chapter 9 for self-hypnosis tools.

- Make sure your hormones are balanced — low estrogen and progesterone in women commonly causes sleep problems. Oral progesterone is better at helping women sleep than other modes of delivery, but you should avoid it or lower your dosage if you feel groggy in the morning.

If you are genuinely adhering to the above recommendations and you still don't sleep soundly, several natural supplements may be helpful. Try taking extra magnesium at dinner or before bed. Magnesium enhances sleep by supporting GABA production (a neurotransmitter that calms the brain) and releasing muscle tension. Many herbs, including valerian root, passionflower, hops, skullcap, lemon balm, catnip, kava kava, and chamomile are also safe and effective sleep aids.

Sleep medications may be helpful but should only be used short-term — they do not treat the underlying cause and you may become dependent on them. However, if you need sleep medications short-term, please use them. I have seen far too many people who haven't slept well, often existing on a few hours of sleep per night for years or decades. After trying many natural options, they often give up due to fear of taking sleep medications. These people are exhausted, depressed, usually overweight, and have significant health problems from years of sleep debt. Although I'm not a fan of using sleep medications (especially since insomnia is often due to an untreated hormone or neurotransmitter imbalance), I strongly urge you to consider using medication for a short while if you are sleep deprived and nothing else works. My sleep-deprived patients are often amazed at how well they feel within a few days simply by getting more sleep! Remember, sleep and exercise are the two panaceas in medicine — if you are to age optimally, you must prioritize doing both every day.

## Step 5: Avoid toxins and do a yearly detox.

This fact is indisputable: we are all toxic. Consider this — the Environmental Protection Agency (EPA) is responsible for a project called "The National Human Adipose Tissue Survey" or NHATS. The purpose of NHATS is to provide data on the amount of dangerous chemicals in the fat tissue of Americans. More than 20 years ago, NHATS reported that 100% of people tested positive for plastics, solvents, and dioxins, and 83% also had significant amounts of PCBs.[132,133] In a more recent study, a nonprofit organization, The Environmental Working Group, identified more than 167 synthetic chemicals and carcinogens in the average US citizen.[134]

It's no surprise that we're all toxic. In the US, more than 1.2 billion pounds of pesticides are used every year[135] — *that's nearly four pounds for every man, woman, and child*. These chemicals can remain in our food — the FDA has found pesticide residue in 50% of domestic fruit and more than 27% of domestic vegetables. Even if we're careful to avoid toxins in our immediate environment, the fact is that we all live "downstream." For example, the EPA maintains a database called the "Toxic Release Inventory" that contains detailed information on nearly 650 chemicals US companies dispose of throughout the year. In 2008, nearly 22,000 facilities reported to the TRI, recording 3.86 billion pounds of chemicals pumped into the air, released into the ground, and dumped into lakes and rivers.[136] These chemicals often end up in the air we breathe, the water we drink, and the food we eat. It's no longer a matter of whether or not you're toxic, it's a matter of how toxic you are and what you're willing to do about it. We are all like Sesame Street's Oscar the Grouch — we live in a garbage can.

So, what can you do? First do your best to avoid exposure to toxins, starting with pesticides. Since most pesticides are fat-soluble and the brain is 60% fat, it's not surprising that research shows an association between pesticide exposure, depression, and neurological diseases such as Parkinson's.[137,138] Pesticides have also been linked to hormone imbalances, and skin, eye, and lung problems.[139-141] The risk for cancer is likely increased with pesticide exposure, with consistent research connecting pesticides to cancers of the brain, pancreas, and prostate.[142-144]

The reason that so many health problems are linked to pesticides is that pesticides are specifically designed to kill living organisms, such as plants, insects, and fungi. Manufacturers of pesticides often defend their products stating that the amount of pesticides on produce is safe due to low concentrations. However, the enormous number of different pesticides coupled with daily exposure can contribute to an overwhelming amount of toxicity in your body.[145] Therefore, it is best to avoid as much pesticide exposure as possible by eating organically grown produce and free-range meat. Although it may be more expensive to eat this way, food is one of the most important investments you can make in your health (remember, food is information for your genes).

The Environmental Working Group's website (www.ewg.org) provides helpful tips about avoiding pesticides. Here's their list, which you can also download as a wallet-sized copy. The "Dirty Dozen" list is in order of the highest pesticide load.

The Dirty Dozen (buy these organic):

- Peaches
- Apples
- Bell peppers
- Celery
- Nectarines
- Strawberries
- Cherries
- Kale
- Lettuce
- Grapes (imported)
- Carrots
- Pears

Clean 15 (lowest in pesticides)

- Onions
- Avocadoes
- Sweet corn
- Pineapple
- Mangoes
- Asparagus
- Sweet peas
- Kiwi
- Cabbage
- Eggplant
- Papaya
- Watermelon
- Broccoli
- Tomatoes
- Sweet potatoes

Besides minimizing pesticide exposure, another step you can take to decrease your toxic load is to avoid xenoestrogens. Xenoestrogens are synthetic chemicals that mimic estrogen in an unhealthy way in the human body. Xenoestrogens disrupt the endocrine system and may increase the risk for brain damage and some cancers. Most insecticides and pesticides are classified as xenoestrogens in addition to chemicals found in plastic. Two of these chemicals, bisphenol-A and phthalates, are known endocrine disruptors and are used in products you use every day.

Bisphenol-A (BPA) is one of the most pervasive chemicals in modern life with more than 2 million tons produced worldwide each year. BPA was originally looked at in the 1930s as a synthetic estrogen replacement,[146] but it was replaced by a similar chemical DES (diethylstilbestrol). DES was taken off the market because daughters born to mothers given DES had a significantly increased risk for breast, vaginal, and cervical cancer.

Bisphenol-A can be found in the epoxy resin lining of cans used for food and soft drinks, and in water bottles, shatterproof baby bottles, and some dental fillings. Most studies on the health effects of BPA have focused on estrogenic activity, but some reports have found that BPA can also cause liver damage.[147,148] In addition, BPA can affect the function of thyroid hormone and the pancreas.[149,150] The US National Health and Nutrition Examination Survey (NHANES) conducted by the Centers for Disease Control and Prevention (CDC) found detectable levels of BPA in 93% of the US population.[151] Recent research suggests that people who drink out of BPA-containing water bottles may substantially increase their total-body BPA level after only one week.[152]

Phthalates are synthetic chemicals added to plastic to increase flexibility. The NHANES study (cited above) measured urinary phthalate metabolites in 2500 people—more than 75% of participants tested positive for phthalates. Phthalates are used in polyvinyl chloride (PVC) products such as vinyl shower curtains, raincoats, cable, flooring, and some plastic toys. The "new car smell" which is especially strong after a car has been sitting in the sun for a few hours, is the smell of phthalates volatilizing from the hot plastic dashboard. The strong chemical odor of a new shower curtain is also due to phthalates.

In men, xenoestrogens such as BPA and phthalates may increase the risk for benign prostatic hyperplasia, prostate cancer, testicular cancer, and low sperm count and motility.[153-155] In women, xenoestrogens may increase the likelihood of developing endometriosis and breast cancer.[156-159] For more information about the link between toxicity and breast cancer, consult the breast cancer fund (www.breastcancerfund.org). A detailed scientific statement presenting "the evidence that endocrine disruptors have effects on male and female reproduction, breast development and cancer, prostate cancer, neuroendocrinology, thyroid, metabolism and obesity, and cardiovascular endocrinology" was recently published by The Endocrine Society.[160] To access a copy of the paper, see: www.endo-society.org/journals/scientificstatements/

You can limit exposure to BPA by never microwaving plastic food containers and avoiding canned food and soft drinks. To decrease exposure in children, do not use plastic baby bottles or infant formulas that come in cans. Plastic containers and water bottles can leach BPA—plastic, marked with the recycling code #7 or the letters "PC," contains BPA. Remember, when buying food in plastic, #7 is not a lucky number. Cloudy-colored plastic and plastics with recycling labels #1, #2, and #4 on the bottom do not contain BPA. Almost all canned food sold in the US has a BPA-based epoxy liner that leaches BPA into the food. The highest concentration is in canned meats, pasta, and soups.[161]  Therefore, eliminating canned food as much as possible can limit BPA exposure. Some forward-thinking companies, such as Eden® Organic, currently offer food in BPA-free cans.

As of July 2008, six phthalates have been banned from children's toys and cosmetics in the US. To limit your exposure to phthalates, make sure your home and car are well ventilated if you smell plastic fumes. *Remember, if you smell chemicals, they're getting into your body.*

Reducing exposure to pesticides and xenoestrogens is critical to maintain hormone balance and promote optimal aging. Since we're all exposed to these harmful chemicals, however, avoiding them as much as possible is not enough. It's important to undergo a yearly detox program to enhance metabolism and excretion of stored toxins. During these 3-4 weeks, pay particular attention to eating an organic, anti-inflammatory, hypoallergenic diet. This means eat organic produce, free-range lean meats or low-mercury containing fish (such as wild salmon, flounder, or arctic cod), and hypoallergenic grains such as rice. During this time, be mindful of drinking at least two liters of clean, filtered water (stored in glass or BPA-free water bottles), and avoid all alcohol, caffeine, and sugar. Many products are available to support your liver and intestines in enhancing metabolism and excretion of toxins. See the Resources section in chapter 9 for more information.

## Step 6: Maintain a healthy weight

Do you avoid looking in the mirror? Do make excuses to yourself about your weight, knowing it's not ideal? If you are overweight, you're in the majority since more than two-thirds of Americans are overweight or obese. If you're not sure whether your weight is ideal, consult the body mass index (www.nhlbisupport.com/bmi) or better yet, have your fat and lean body mass percentages measured via bioelectrical impendence analysis (BIA). A BIA machine works by passing a small electrical current through the body to measure resistance. Because lean body mass (which includes muscle, bone, and organs) and fat conduct the current differently, they can be measured through BIA.

There are many contributing factors to being overweight, including stress, lack of exercise, poor diet choices, and hormone imbalances. Genetics may play a role; however, as you learned in chapter one, how your genes express themselves is largely within your control—influenced by your diet, lifestyle, nutrient intake, and toxicity level.

Perhaps you've heard that weight gain is common with aging due to the overall slowing of metabolism. It is true that after age 45 the average person loses 10% of their muscle mass per decade.[162] This equates to losing one-third to one-half pound of muscle each year, and gaining that much fat. Because muscle burns more calories compared to fat, the total calories you burn each day also declines with aging.

The good news is that aerobic exercise and weight lifting can offset the decline in metabolism associated with aging.[163,164] Restoring hormones to youthful levels with bioidentical hormones can improve muscle and bone mass. In addition, supplementing with fish oil and coenzyme Q10 may help—fish oil promotes insulin sensitivity and coenzyme Q10 enables mitochondria to make ATP for optimal energy levels and metabolism.

If you are overweight, commit to a plan to reduce it. Nearly all studies show that eating a calorie-restricted diet high in nutrients can slow signs of aging, including telomere shortening, as well as lead to weight loss.[165-168] No single diet is best for everyone. In fact, a recent long-term study that compared diets with different compositions of fat, protein, and carbohydrates, showed that weight loss was related to calories, not which macronutrient (fat, protein, or carbs) was emphasized.[169] When it comes to carbohydrates, however, eating those with a low glycemic index does lead to greater weight loss.[170]

The most successful weight loss programs combine changes in behavior, diet, nutritional education, and exercise.[171] In other words, just following a diet is usually not enough to maintain weight loss — it's more effective to learn about nutrition, improve your food choices, implement more exercise, and enhance self-awareness about why you eat the way you do. In addition, accountability — either through frequent group attendance or individual sessions — leads to a much better likelihood of achieving weight loss goals.[172] If you want to achieve and maintain your ideal weight, here is a foolproof plan that will work:

- Record what you eat and your calorie intake. You must measure your food to be accurate — most people under-report portion sizes.

- Reduce your calories by 500-750 calories per day; this will lead to a healthy weight loss of 1-2 pounds per week.

- Learn about nutrition and healthy food choices.

- Adopt new behavior regarding food (e.g., become aware of "emotional eating").

- Exercise regularly.

- Report your progress to a group or individual coach to enhance accountability.

If you've tried unsuccessfully to lose weight on your own in the past, consider investing in a program such as Weight Watchers,® or hiring a Certified Life Coach. If you do decide to decrease your calorie intake, please do not eat a very low calorie diet (under 800 calories per day) without medical supervision.

## Step 7: Supplements.

Notice that this step is number 7 in "The 8 Steps for Achieving HormoneSynergy." This is because supplements should be used in addition to, not in place of, the previous steps. In my practice I've seen many patients come in with a shopping bag or tackle box full of pills, proudly showcasing the huge number of supplements they take. Many supplement takers eat an unhealthy diet, skimp on sleep, remain sedentary, and live high stress lives. I'm dismayed that people think taking pills, natural or pharmaceutical, is a reasonable substitute for a healthy lifestyle and life-affirming diet. Therefore, if you're hoping to find the magic herbs or nutrients that will enable you to skip the previous steps, you'll be disappointed to know there aren't any. If you're already following the first 6 steps as much as possible, there are exceptional quality supplements, often referred to as "nutraceuticals," that can certainly help in your quest to attain hormone balance and optimal aging.

## What to look for when purchasing supplements

It's important to keep in mind that not all products are alike, no matter what the manufacturer or label may claim. Make sure the supplements you take are made in facilities that have pharmaceutical certification or are certified for good manufacturing practices (GMP) by the NPA (Natural Products Association), NSF (National Sanitation Foundation International), or TGA (Therapeutic Goods Administration of Australia). This certification ensures that the products you use are of exceptional quality.

Besides coming from GMP-certified companies, ideally the supplements you take should be scientifically evaluated to verify the presence and concentration of active constituents. Few supplement manufacturers conduct clinical trials on their formulas to document safety and effectiveness. This is because research is very expensive to perform. However, purchasing supplements that are documented for safety and effectiveness is a reliable investment in your health.

In addition to quality assurance and evaluation via clinical trials, look for bioavailable forms of nutrients and dosages. Consider the supplements you take to be as important as any medications prescribed by your doctor. In fact, you may consider them to be more important than medications since they can help you prevent the "polypharmacy" that is standard of care for aging Americans (remember, 25% of all Medicare patients use six or more drugs every day). The Resources section in chapter 9 lists exceptional supplement manufacturers.

## Multiple vitamin and mineral formula

Vitamins and minerals play vital roles in all body processes. Taking a multiple vitamin and mineral formula ensures adequate intake of micronutrients not always found in high enough amounts in your diet. Your multi is nutritional insurance for health maintenance and disease prevention.

Ideally, your multi should contain the most bioavailable, active forms of nutrients. For example, calcium citrate, ascorbate, or malate are more absorbable than the cheaper version, calcium carbonate (which is chalk). Natural vitamin E (d-alpha-tocopherol) or mixed tocopherols are the forms the body needs, not cheaper, synthetic dl-alpha-tocopherol. Bioavailable vitamin B6 (pyridoxal-5-phosphate) and folic acid (L-methylfolate or 5-methyl-tetrahydrofolate) are much better at performing cellular functions than other forms. Methylcobalamin, the active form of B12, is a superior form compared to cheaper cyanocobalamin, which contains a cyanide group. It may be beneficial to take a multi that has extra B5 (pantothenic acid), B6, and vitamin C, since these nutrients are critical for normal adrenal gland function and recovery from stress.

## Antioxidants

Free radical damage and oxidative stress accelerate aging of your cells. Antioxidants are substances that neutralize free radicals — in other words, antioxidants stop the chain reaction of electron stealing. Some, such as the enzymes superoxide dismutase, catalase, and glutathione peroxidase, are made by your body; other antioxidants are consumed through your diet or via supplements. These include beta-carotene and other carotenoids, vitamins A, C, and E, and the mineral selenium (technically, selenium isn't an antioxidant; it's an important component of antioxidant enzymes). In addition, substances such as lutein (the yellow pigment in corn or squash, or dark green color in vegetables), lycopene (from tomatoes and grapefruit), and flavonoids and polyphenols (found in colored food such as berries, grapes, and red wine) have the ability to stop free radical damage.

Many exceptional quality multivitamin and mineral formulas contain antioxidants. Since you now understand the value of eating at least 5-7 servings of vegetables and fruit per day (where you'll get loads of antioxidants), you can add an antioxidant supplement if your multi doesn't contain one, or consider drinking a powdered green drink daily to minimize free radical damage and cellular aging.

## Coenzyme Q10

Coenzyme Q10 (or "CoQ10") is an enzyme used for ATP production in mitochondria. Your life depends on ATP for normal cellular function and nearly all the energy generated by your cells requires CoQ10 for production. CoQ10 is also a potent antioxidant that prevents "internal rusting" of your cells.[173]

CoQ10 levels decrease with age[174], and can significantly decline (up to 40%) with the use of statin (cholesterol-lowering) medication.[175] CoQ10 is most important for your heart, liver, and brain, since these organs have a high-energy demand. CoQ10 supplementation may prevent DNA damage that contributes to age-related conditions, and may protect against heart disease, cancer, diabetes, and brain disorders such as Alzheimer's. [176-180]

Although no human studies have shown that taking CoQ10 prolongs life, it seems reasonable to supplement with CoQ10 for prevention of age-related CoQ10 decline in the mitochondria. If you've been diagnosed with conditions such as heart disease, cardiomyopathy, arrhythmias, or heart failure, it's even more important that you supplement with CoQ10. Since CoQ10 has been shown to be low in people with muscular dystrophies, Parkinson's disease, cancer, diabetes, kidney disease, and HIV/AIDs, taking CoQ10 if you have any of these conditions is important.

The dosage and form of CoQ10 you should take depends upon your condition and age. Most research shows that dosages of 100 to 600 mg of CoQ10 (ubiquinone) is needed per day for beneficial effects, or 50 to 300 mg of the reduced form of CoQ10 (ubiquinol). Ubiquinol is the most predominant form of CoQ10 in the body. Although ubiquinone can be converted into ubiquinol, a recent study suggests that this conversion declines with aging and it may be more beneficial to supplement with ubiquinol.[181] Whatever form of CoQ10 you take, make sure the manufacturer can prove its product raises CoQ10 levels in the human body.

## Fish Oil

Fish oil contains the omega-3 essential fatty acids EPA (eicosapentaenoic acid) and DHA (docosahexaenoic acid). These fats are "essential" because they cannot be made by your body — they must come from your diet. The EPA and DHA in fish oil are crucial for healthy nerve and brain function. In addition, EPA and DHA ensure normal blood pressure, cholesterol, and insulin levels, and keep pain and inflammation low. Taking fish oil can decrease your risk for a heart attack or stroke, prevent diabetes, treat depression and anxiety, and prevent neurodegenerative diseases such as Parkinson's and Alzheimer's.[182-187] People with heart disease who have higher levels of EPA and DHA have been shown to have slower rates of telomere shortening.[188] Therefore, supplementing with fish oil may actually delay the aging of your cells. Because of its benefits in nearly all body systems, fish oil is one of the most important supplements you can take.

Make sure the fish oil you use is of exceptional quality. The pharmaceutical giant, GlaxoSmithKline, has developed a concentrated fish oil called Lovaza®, which contains approximately 465 mg EPA and 375 mg DHA per capsule. Lovaza is very expensive, costing between $150 and $200 for 100 capsules. Several supplement manufacturers have excellent quality fish oil that has been tested, preferably before and after production, for heavy metals such as mercury and arsenic, PCBs, and dioxins. The cost for these products is considerably less than pharmaceutical fish oil.

Fish oil dosage should be based on your current health, ranging from 500 to 4,000 mg of EPA and DHA per day. If you have an inflammatory or neurological condition, or high triglycerides, you may benefit from the higher dosages. Note: fish oil can thin your blood; therefore, if you will be undergoing surgery in the next few weeks, or if you're on a blood thinning medication, please talk to your doctor before taking fish oil.

## Vitamin D₃

People with higher levels of vitamin D age more slowly than those with lower levels. This is likely related to vitamin D enhancing the length of telomeres and inhibiting inflammation.[189-191]

Vitamin D plays a role in the health of numerous parts of the body including the brain, heart, skin, ovaries, breasts, testes, and prostate. Vitamin D is also necessary for maintaining strong bones and muscles—in fact, a deficiency of vitamin D can cause muscle and bone pain.[192] Optimal vitamin D levels may reduce your risk for several health problems including autoimmune diseases, depression, cognitive decline, high blood pressure, cardiovascular disease, and diabetes.[193-197] Vitamin D may also prevent cancer—research on cancer prevention and vitamin D levels is strongest for cancers of the breast prostate, and colon. [198-202]

Your skin makes vitamin D from sun exposure. Unfortunately, however, the skin becomes less efficient at producing vitamin D as you age. If you take vitamin D supplements, ideally your dosage should be based on lab testing. Taking 1000 to 2000 IU of vitamin $D_3$ or cholecalciferol daily, may be adequate—although people with low blood levels may need a significantly higher dosage. It's important to note that too much vitamin D can lead to kidney stones and calcification of soft tissue. In addition, anyone with primary hyperparathyroidism should not take vitamin D supplements.

## Resveratrol

Rarely has a nutritional supplement caused as much enthusiasm from optimal aging physicians, as well as false claims from unscientific, unscrupulous companies trying to make quick money, as resveratrol. Resveratrol is a compound found in red wine and is made by grapes and other plants in response to fungal infection. In the past decade there have literally been thousands of studies aimed at determining how grapes, wine, and resveratrol may be beneficial for prevention and treatment of diseases of aging, especially regarding cancer, type 2 diabetes, cardiovascular disease, and neurological conditions.[203]

Research in fish has shown that resveratrol significantly increases life span and slows brain deterioration.[204] In mice, resveratrol has been shown to lengthen life span through a mechanism similar to calorie restriction.[205] Evidence also exists that resveratrol increases nitric oxide to dilate blood vessels and lower blood pressure, and that it decreases the stickiness of blood, reducing the possibility of blood clots and strokes.[206-208]

Resveratrol is a powerful antioxidant that can help prevent free radical damage to the brain and promote normal DNA replication.[209] Although performed in vitro (which means in a laboratory), there are many studies revealing how resveratrol can prevent or treat cancer.[210]

Since resveratrol seems safe even at high dosages,[211] it's likely good optimal aging insurance to include it in your supplement plan. Make sure the resveratrol you purchase is *trans*-resveratrol (rather than *cis*-resveratrol). The most beneficial dosage hasn't been established but is likely a minimum of 100 to 200 mg per day.

## Indole-3-carbinol

Indole-3-carbinol (I3C) is a potent phytochemical found in cruciferous vegetables such as cabbage, cauliflower, broccoli, turnips, kale, and Brussels sprouts. Research on I3C suggests that it may prevent breast, uterine, and cervical cancers in women, and prostate cancer in men.[212-216] This is likely due to the ability of I3C to increase the ratio of 2-hydroxyestrone to 16-alpha-hydroxyestrone metabolites of estrogen.[217-221] The 2-hydroxy metabolites of estrogen have weak activity, whereas the 16-alpha-hydroxy metabolites have persistent estrogenic activity, promoting proliferation of cells.

Most studies that show beneficial effects of indole-3-carbinol have used 200 to 600 mg per day. People who weigh more than 180 pounds, or who have high 16-hydroxyestrogen levels (measurable via urine or blood testing) may need higher dosages, up to 800 mg per day.

# Chapter 7: Bioidentical hormone replacement

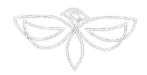

Humans are a unique species when it comes to the fact that we live much of our lives outside our reproductive years. Most animals in the wild do not live beyond their ability to reproduce—many don't even live beyond puberty. Our species' increased life expectancy is relatively recent—only in the past few generations has it extended beyond 60 years.

There is much controversy about whether or not it's appropriate to restore hormones to youthful levels as people age. This chapter will discuss what bioidentical hormones are, safety information, research, and resources for learning more to determine whether bioidentical hormone replacement is right for you.

In this book, the term "bioidentical" refers to the molecular structure of a hormone—this is not the same as the term "natural." For example, Premarin®, which comes from pregnant mare's urine, could be considered "natural," however, it is not structurally identical to human estrogen (although it would be bioidentical if you were a pregnant horse!) The same is true for Provera®, a synthetic progestin that has been shown to have significant detrimental health effects. When the term bioidentical hormone replacement therapy or BHRT is used in this section, it refers to <u>human-identical</u> hormones.

When discussing bioidentical hormone replacement, it's essential to separate fact from opinion. (To access a copy of Dr. Retzler's "BHRT Position Paper" as well as references for research on bioidentical hormones, please see www.hormonesynergy.com.)

## Facts

The following **facts** should be considered before choosing to supplement with hormones:

- Many women and men have significant symptoms as they age. No two people are identical in terms of their hormone production or the symptoms they experience.

- The foundation for preventing and managing hormone-related symptoms includes eating a healthy diet, exercising regularly, minimizing stress, and avoiding environmental toxins.

- If symptoms persist, hormone replacement is an option that carries both benefits and risks.

- People have different medication needs and drug detoxifying capacities. Testing may help determine appropriate, individualized dosages.

- Synthetic hormones (notably Premarin,® Provera,® and methyltestosterone, a synthetic testosterone found in Estratest® and Syntest®) have been shown to have serious negative health consequences including an increased risk for breast cancer, blood clots, heart disease, and stroke. Synthetic oral testosterone has been shown to increase the risk for liver inflammation and liver cancer in men. Due to liver toxicity, methyltestosterone has been taken off the market for men, but (in lower dosages) is still given to women in Estratest® and Syntest.®

## Safety of BHRT

There is a large body of research involving the effectiveness of bioidentical estradiol, progesterone, and testosterone (for a look at the research, see the references available at www.hormonesynergy.com.) Bioidentical hormones do carry risks, especially when administered in excessive dosages, outside of physiological levels; overall, however, compared to synthetic hormones, their risk profile is lower. This is especially true for progesterone vs. progestins, and testosterone versus methyltestosterone. More research about long-term effects of bioidentical hormones still needs to be done.

Many FDA-approved medications contain bioidentical hormones (e.g., bioidentical estradiol patches such as Climara® or Vivelle®, bioidentical progesterone such as Prometrium® and Crinone®, and bioidentical testosterone such as Androderm®, Androgel®, or Testopel®). Bioidentical hormones can also be made as individual preparations by compounding pharmacists. Compounded medications have been available since the 1930s. Organizations such as the Professional Compounding Centers of America (PCCA) provide continuing education seminars for pharmacists and physicians, as well as a source of FDA-approved ingredients subjected to rigorous quality assurance standards.

## *Opinions*

Following are some **opinions** that make sense when putting together a treatment plan using BHRT:

- It makes sense to test baseline hormone production. If low levels or hormone-related symptoms indicate it to be necessary, it also seems reasonable to supplement with bioidentical hormones as long as levels are not above physiological range (youthful levels). There is no established protocol for such treatment and potential risks do exist.

- It is your right and responsibility to choose an experienced physician who listens, provides you with information, and respects your treatment decisions. Treating hormone imbalances requires a comprehensive understanding of endocrinology and gynecology, as well as significant clinical experience. It is impossible for any physician to be an expert in all areas of health. Treat your health care providers as teachers or consultants, and recognize that each member of your health care team may have different experience and knowledge. Expect your physician to provide you with information on available research, benefits, and risks of any treatment you choose. Do not be afraid to question any treatment or to make your own healthcare decisions. If your healthcare provider is unaware of research about bioidentical hormones, he or she may sincerely—yet mistakenly—say there is no research, or that bioidentical hormones are dangerous. You may want to give your doctor a copy of this book, direct him or her to the references on the HormoneSynergy website, or you may want to find another doctor to help with this area of your health.

## *BHRT Options*

There are many options for supplementing with bioidentical estradiol, progesterone, and testosterone. If needed, there are options for replacing thyroid hormone, DHEA, and cortisol. Finding the ideal dosages and delivery methods of bioidentical hormones for your body may take some time and adjustments. This may require laboratory testing or several visits with your healthcare provider. Once your bioidentical hormone treatment regimen is decided, it's important to see your doctor if new symptoms develop, and to visit at least once every year to discuss your health status, make sure dosages are still optimal, and review any new research findings that impact your health or decisions.

If you do choose to use compounded bioidentical hormones rather than FDA-approved pharmaceuticals, please know that not all compounding pharmacies are equal. For example, in 2001 the FDA tested 29 products from 12 compounding pharmacies that allowed products to be ordered over the Internet.[222] Many different types of medications (including hormones) and different modes of delivery (including sterile injectables, pellet implants, and oral capsules) were tested. Of the 29 products, ten failed testing for potency; in these cases, the amount of active ingredients were lower than the label listed. Thankfully, none of the injectable products or pellet implants failed sterility testing.

Compounding pharmacies are regulated by individual states, not by the Food and Drug Administration (FDA). Ideally, the compounding pharmacy you use should be accredited by the Pharmacy Compounding Accreditation Board (PCAB). PCAB certification provides assurance to consumers that a pharmacy has demonstrated superior quality and safety in compounding practices. Compounding pharmacies can vary in terms of the expertise of the pharmacist making your medication, quality control, customer service, and price. Make sure your compounding pharmacy is PCAB accredited, even if their products are more expensive — your health and safety are worth it.

The rest of this section provides a general overview of the different modes of delivery for bioidentical estrogens, progesterone, and testosterone, as well as a brief description of the pros and cons of each delivery method. A short section on thyroid hormone is also provided. Please note that this information is meant to be general — hormone dosages and detailed prescribing information is beyond the scope of this book.

## Bioidentical Estrogens

Bioidentical estrogen supplementation options include oral capsules or tablets, sublingual troches (lozenges dissolved in the mouth), transdermal (through the skin) weekly or twice-a-week patches, topical or intravaginal creams, or estradiol pellet implants. There are pros and cons to each delivery method so it's important to consider them individually.

Oral estrogens can be effective at managing symptoms but they also increase the risk for blood clots — this is true for synthetic as well as bioidentical oral estrogens.[223] In addition, oral estradiol promotes a ratio of estrogens (more estrone than estradiol) that is not the same as women make prior to menopause (premenopausal women have a ratio of estradiol to estrone of 2:1). Therefore, oral estrogen replacement should be used as a last resort since other equally effective, safer modes of delivery are available.

Sublingual troches or lozenges can be made by a compounding pharmacy and dissolved between the cheek and gum or under the tongue to provide quick relief. Women with occasional hot flashes or menstrual migraines often benefit from this mode of delivery. In my clinical practice, I've noticed women with sleep problems and depression sometimes respond better to the troche delivery of estrogen. Troches may need to be used more than once a day to be effective, and they may not deliver steady levels of estradiol. In addition, care must be taken to avoid swallowing the estradiol in troches.

Transdermal patches (similar to a band-aid or "film" applied to the buttocks, belly, or hip area) can provide low-dose, steady delivery of bioidentical estradiol without the increased risk of blood clots seen with oral preparations.[224,225] Occasionally, women may have skin irritation from patches, although the twice-a-week, smaller patches (such as the Vivelle dot®) tend to be well tolerated. If you use a patch, make sure it contains only estradiol since all combination patches contain synthetic progestins.

Vaginal administration of hormones can be effective since the cells of the vagina are very good at absorbing fat-soluble hormones.[226] Intravaginal estrogen preparations can resolve vaginal dryness and urinary symptoms, and are likely the safest form of estrogen replacement. Estriol, a weak estrogen, is quite effective at treating vaginal dryness, does not increase breast cancer risk,[227-231] and can safely be used by breast cancer survivors.[232]

In some women, intravaginal estrogens may resolve systemic symptoms such as hot flashes, night sweats, decreased memory, or mood problems.[233] Intravaginal estradiol preparations are available in pharmaceutical, bioidentical form. In addition, vaginal creams can be compounded to individualized dosages and concentrations. Compounding can allow for more concentrated cream; in this case less cream would be needed, preventing it from being messy.

Topical estrogen creams and gels are found in the pharmaceuticals Estrasorb®, Estrogel®, Elestrin®, Divigel®, and the spray, Evamist®; creams and gels can also be compounded to individualized dosages. Topical estrogens can be used once or twice per day and many women find them effective. In some women, topical estrogens vary in absorption, causing fluctuating hormone levels. Since creams or gels can rub off on spouses, other family members, and pets, it's important to be careful when using topical hormone preparations. Topical estrogen creams or gels can be used if intravaginal or patch estrogens aren't effective, or if a woman doesn't want to use those administration methods.

Subcutaneous pellet implants are an effective, hassle-free way to supplement with bioidentical estradiol. Pellets are implanted in the fat tissue of the hip or abdomen, last approximately 4-6 months, and result in a steady delivery of hormone. However, women with an intact uterus (i.e., women who haven't had a hysterectomy) are more likely to experience bleeding with estradiol pellets than with other forms of estrogen replacement.

The goals for most women using estrogen replacement are to provide symptom relief, to promote brain, bone, and cardiovascular protection, and to keep skin and vaginal tissue healthy. This can nearly always be accomplished without monthly bleeding. Any bleeding in a menopausal woman may be a sign of a uterine problem, including uterine cancer. It's crucial to see your physician if you experience bleeding after menopause, whether or not you use bioidentical estrogen replacement therapy. In addition, progesterone supplementation is necessary if you use estrogen replacement (except for intravaginal estriol or low-dose, intravaginal estradiol) since it protects the uterus. A woman who uses estrogen replacement must use progesterone at least 12 days per month to lower her risk for uterine cancer.

It's essential to note that not all women need estrogen replacement therapy. Some women age gracefully by following the previous 7 steps to achieving HormoneSynergy, and some women need only progesterone, DHEA, or testosterone supplementation to feel their best. Bioidentical testosterone can convert into estradiol in many tissues, including the brain, heart, and bones,[234] and may be as effective as estrogen replacement for some women.[235]

### *Bioidentical Progesterone*

Bioidentical progesterone is <u>not</u> the same as synthetic progestins (such as Provera®), and does not create the same increased risk for blood clots[236] or breast cancer as synthetic progestins.[237,238] Bioidentical progesterone can be used orally, topically, or intravaginally. If a woman with a uterus takes estrogen, she <u>must</u> use progesterone at least 12 days per month to lower her risk for uterine cancer.

<u>Oral progesterone</u> can be taken as a pharmaceutical (Prometrium®), which is micronized progesterone in peanut oil, or it can be compounded to individualized dosages in a sustained-release format. Oral progesterone can be a good choice for women who have sleep problems or anxiety since one of the metabolites of oral progesterone, 5-allopregnanolone, binds to GABA receptors in the brain[239] (GABA is a calming neurotransmitter).

<u>Topical or intravaginal progesterone cream</u>, which is usually compounded in a hypo-allergenic base, is very effective at managing PMS, fibrocystic breast changes, breast tenderness, and menstrual cramps. If a woman uses estrogen replacement, topical progesterone may not be as effective at protecting the uterus as oral or vaginal progesterone; however, two small studies have shown that topical progesterone can protect the uterus.[240,241]

Do not use progesterone every day if you're still having periods (best to discuss this with a knowledgeable doctor to find out the right dosage and frequency for you). Progesterone supplementation can sometimes help with menopausal symptoms without the need for estrogen.[242,243]

## *Bioidentical Testosterone*

Supplementing with bioidentical testosterone has been shown to offer many benefits for women and men. For example, testosterone enhances libido, or sex drive in both sexes.[244-246]  It also improves overall sense of well-being and alleviates depression.[247,248]  As you learned in chapter two, testosterone is very important for brain health—if your level is low, you may be at an increased risk for developing dementia and Alzheimer's.[249,250]

Testosterone supplementation may also prevent cardiovascular disease since it improves the health of the heart and blood vessels, and lowers bad (LDL) cholesterol.[251-253] Lean body mass improves with testosterone supplementation since testosterone increases muscle mass and strength and decreases fat tissue in both women and men.[254-256] Lastly, testosterone supplementation can reverse bone loss—in studies where women received estrogen and testosterone, bone density improved, whereas women who received estrogen alone merely maintained their bone density.[257,258]

**For men,** bioidentical testosterone is available in many forms including compounded sublingual troches or lozenges, a pharmaceutical tablet that adheres to the gums (Striant®), topical creams or gels, transdermal (through the skin) patches, or pellet implants.

**Options for women** include compounded creams or gels (used topically or intravaginally), or pellet implants. Currently the only FDA-approved medication for women is synthetic, methyltestosterone, which has been shown to increase hepatitis and liver cancer in men. Therefore, all forms of bioidentical testosterone must be individually compounded for women. Oral testosterone is never a good option for anyone since it may cause liver problems and other forms of testosterone are safer and more effective.

Topical creams or gels can be compounded to individualized dosages for both women and men. The pharmaceutical gels, Androgel® and Testim,® are available for men only. Creams and gels are rubbed into the shoulder or non-hairy parts of the chest in men, and into the inner arms, wrists, or backs of the knees, in women. Women may also find that inserting testosterone cream vaginally leads to excellent absorption and results. In men, topical testosterone causes significantly less skin reactions than patches. Showering or bathing must be avoided for several hours after application to ensure adequate absorption. In addition, care must be taken to avoid possible transfer of testosterone to partners, family members, or pets.

The transdermal patch (Androderm®) for men is applied to the back, abdomen, or upper arm each night. The application site must be rotated to decrease skin reaction; unfortunately, skin irritation is very common with this mode of delivery. Transdermal patches do not usually achieve high serum testosterone levels, although men may prefer them to the gel due to the decreased risk of transferring testosterone to others.

Sublingual troches or lozenges are dissolved between the cheek and gum or under the tongue, and must be formulated by a compounding pharmacist. Troches can produce very good blood levels of testosterone, although they often need to be used twice a day. Testosterone troches may cause a rapid rise in testosterone, leading to agitation or anxiety in some men. In addition, rapid elevations of testosterone can increase estradiol production due to aromatization. Care must be taken to dissolve the troche between the cheek and gum or under the tongue, rather than swallowed. Liver enzymes should be monitored in men using sublingual troches since oral (swallowed) testosterone can have detrimental effects on the liver.

The buccal tablet called Striant® is a new form of testosterone replacement for men that consists of applying a tablet to the gums, where it forms a putty-like substance, twice per day. The testosterone in Striant is absorbed directly into the bloodstream, which is safer than oral (swallowed) testosterone. Some men may experience gum irritation with this mode of delivery, and, unfortunately, it is expensive if you must pay out-of-pocket.

Testosterone pellets can be implanted in the hip or abdomen in both women and men every 4-6 months. When compared to other forms of testosterone replacement, pellets provide stable, optimal levels of testosterone; some studies have shown that men prefer testosterone pellets compared to other forms of testosterone replacement.[259-262] Pellets only need to be implanted 2-3 times a year for women and men, and they avoid the problem of transference to others as seen with topical applications.

## More about subcutaneous hormone pellets

Although bioidentical hormone pellets have been used since the late 1930s and are the oldest form of BHRT,[263] many physicians are unaware that they exist. This is, in part, due to lack of FDA-approval for pellets in women (Testopel® testosterone pellets are FDA-approved for men). This is also due to the source of continuing medical education for physicians—doctors get much of their continuing education from drug companies, and the makers of FDA-approved hormones have a huge profit incentive in teaching doctors about their products.

Many patients find bioidentical hormone pellets the most effective form of BHRT—in terms of symptom improvement, and in terms of convenience, since pellets only need to be inserted 2-3 times a year.[264-267]

Pellets are available as compounded estradiol and testosterone for women, or compounded testosterone or the FDA-approved Testopel® pellet for men. Since they are implanted in fat tissue, pellets provide consistent, stable levels of hormones; in other words, they avoid the fluctuations, or ups and downs, and absorption problems seen with other methods of hormone delivery.

Studies regarding pellets and breast cancer risk in women have been favorable. One 18-year study of 261 women in the Netherlands, showed that estradiol pellets did not increase breast cancer risk.[268] In another Australian study that looked at testosterone pellets along with usual hormone replacement, testosterone negated the increased risk of breast cancer from HRT (meaning the women who received testosterone pellets had a lower than expected risk for breast cancer).[269] Two studies of breast cancer survivors noted no increased risk of cancer recurrence or death with estradiol pellets, testosterone pellets, or both.[270,271]

Although many doctors are unaware of pellets, estradiol and/or testosterone pellets are a very effective delivery system to maintain and reverse bone loss; in several studies, pellets have even been shown to be superior to other forms of HRT regarding bone health.[272-286]

In women, estradiol pellets have been shown to help with migraines and menstrual headaches.[287] Overall, estradiol and testosterone pellets can alleviate menopausal symptoms including hot flashes, heart palpitations, and insomnia. Sexual problems such as loss of libido and painful intercourse are successfully treated with pellets. Lastly, pellets have been shown to reverse fatigue, depression, irritability, poor memory, and decreased concentration in women.[288-293]

In men and women, testosterone pellets have been shown to improve energy, alleviate depression and anxiety, and increase sense of well-being. Estradiol and testosterone pellets can lower LDL (bad) and raise HDL (good) cholesterol levels, and protect the heart by enhancing the health of blood vessels.[294-296]

There are 2 downsides to using pellets in women. The first is that estradiol (not testosterone) pellets are more likely to cause bleeding in a woman who still has her uterus when compared to other forms of estrogen replacement. This may be dose related (in other words, higher dosages are more likely to cause the uterine lining to build up, leading to bleeding). The second downside to pellets is that they're difficult to remove — this concern can be alleviated by making sure your physician is very familiar with pellet dosages, the research on pellets, and with evaluating you based on lab results and your individual symptoms, risks, and health goals.

## Thyroid hormone

It may be surprising to learn that all thyroid hormone medications are bioidentical — whether synthetic (such as Synthroid®) or of animal thyroid gland origin (such as Armour® thyroid or Nature-throid®). This means that all thyroid medications contain human-identical hormone. All thyroid hormone must be bioidentical because every cell of your body needs thyroid hormone, and it must fit its receptor exactly for proper activity. The main difference between thyroid preparations is that some contain only T4 (mainly inactive thyroid) and some contain T3 (active thyroid hormone). The "standard of care" is to prescribe only medications containing T4, with the assumption that the T4 will be converted to active T3. However the conversion of T4 to T3 can be prevented by stress and high cortisol levels, zinc or selenium deficiency, and excess mercury. This will leave people with symptoms of low thyroid, even though lab results (such as TSH or T4 levels) are within the reference range.

Some people with low-thyroid symptoms or lab results need only T4, others need T4 combined with T3, while others need only T3. Options for T4 include Synthroid®, Levothyroxine®, and Levothroid®;

options for combined T4/T3 include Armour®, Nature-throid®, Thyrolar®, and Westhroid.® The option that most mimics the natural production of thyroid is to first supplement with T4 only. Once your TSH level is ideal (for most individuals this will be between 0.3 and 2.0 μIU/L), you can measure your free T3 level (optimal is >300 pg/dL)—if your T3 is suboptimal, your physician can prescribe the pharmaceutical Cytomel® or compounded, sustained-release T3. The benefit of compounded thyroid is that it can be made as a sustained-release capsule, to be taken once or twice a day. This mode of delivery best mimics what your body's own thyroid production would be.

# Chapter 8: Breast Cancer and Prostate Cancer

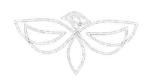

Breast cancer is the most frequently diagnosed cancer in women. A woman's risk for breast cancer increases with age. Currently, a woman has approximately a 12% chance of developing breast cancer if she lives to be 90 years old; this also means her risk of not getting breast cancer is approximately 88%. Death rates from breast cancer have decreased since 1990. There were more than 180,000 cases of invasive breast cancer diagnosed in the US in 2008 with 40,000 deaths. Breast cancer is the second leading cause of cancer deaths — lung cancer is the first. To some extent, breast cancer may be preventable.

Cancer occurs when cells divide and grow without restraint. The growth and death of cells is usually regulated; however, when normal cell regulators malfunction and cells don't die at the proper rate, they continue to divide, and cancer can develop.

Breast cancer usually grows slowly. By the time a tumor is large enough to be felt as a lump, it may have been growing for 10 years and the spread of tumor cells (metastasis) may have already occurred. Therefore, screening methods such as mammography, ultrasound, MRI, or thermography, are important tools in providing early detection. In addition, preventive measures such as a healthy diet and lifestyle, nutritional supplementation, and exercise are crucial.

Knowing the risk factors for breast cancer can help you identify your specific risk. Breast cancer risk factors can be categorized as "modifiable" and "non-modifiable." Although non-modifiable risk factors cannot be altered, modifiable risk factors can be changed based on daily choices regarding diet, exercise, lifestyle habits, and stress management.

Non-modifiable risk factors for breast cancer include:

- Being female
- Advancing age
- Family history (mother, sister, or positive BRCA1 or BRCA2 gene mutation)
- Early menarche (first menstrual period)
- Late menopause
- Diethylstilbestrol (DES) use by mother

Modifiable risk factors for breast cancer include:

- Obesity
- Lack of exercise
- Hormones: conventional HRT—synthetic progestins and, possibly, synthetic estrogens, depending on duration of use; birth control pills (some studies show this, some don't); bioidentical estrogen (depending on duration of use)
- Poor diet: high animal and trans fats, low fiber intake, deficient intake of fruits and vegetables
- Breast trauma
- Late age pregnancy, never having been pregnant, lack of breast feeding
- High alcohol intake (>1 drink per day)
- Cigarette smoking
- Working the "graveyard" shift
- Environmental toxin exposure (radiation, xenoestrogens, second hand smoke)
- Benign breast disease (fibrocystic breast changes, may or may not increase risk)

### Breast cancer and hormones

Currently every 50-year-old woman has about a 2.8% chance of developing breast cancer by age 60. This translates to an absolute risk of 2.8 breast cancer cases out of 100 women.

Most studies show the overall risk of developing breast cancer is higher with the use of synthetic estrogens and synthetic progestins. That means out of 100 women age 50 using synthetic hormone replacement (according to the Women's Health Initiative data), the number who will develop breast cancer by age 60 is 3.5. What this means is that per 100 women who use synthetic estrogen and synthetic progestin (Prempro®) slightly less than one extra woman will develop breast cancer. That increase, from 2.8 to 3.5 per 100 women, represents a 25% increase in risk.

For comparison to other risk factors, some studies show obesity and high insulin levels can cause the risk for breast cancer to go up 200 to 300%.[297-299] In addition, some antibiotics used for more than 500 days in a lifetime, or more than 25 prescriptions over 17 years, can increase the risk by 150% to 200%.[300,301]

When evaluating information regarding hormone use and breast cancer risk, it's imperative to determine

- what hormone is being discussed
  - synthetic estrogen versus bioidentical estradiol or estriol
  - synthetic progestins versus bioidentical progesterone
  - synthetic methyltestosterone versus bioidentical testosterone
- mode of delivery
  - oral
  - transdermal
  - topical
  - pellet
  - vaginal

as the risk varies across these variables. In addition, risk varies based on the number of years of hormone use. Not enough studies have been performed using individualized dosages of compounded hormones (based on lab testing, clinical assessment, and risk factors) since most studies use uniform modes of delivery and dosages of hormones for all women. However, one recently published small study of 189 women reported no increased risk of breast cancer, blood clots, or strokes with bioidentical hormones that were prescribed based on individualized dosages (determined via blood testing and symptom control). Women in this study were monitored for one to three years, and most had significant improvements in menopausal symptoms.[302]

The following summary is meant to give you succinct information based on available research regarding estrogens, progestins and progesterone, and testosterone with regard to breast cancer risk.

**Estrogens,** especially estradiol and estrone, stimulate proliferation of both breast tissue and breast cancer cells. There is much confusion about the use of estrogen replacement therapy (ERT) and breast cancer risk; this is true for the use of bioidentical estrogens as well as synthetic forms, such as Premarin. It's helpful to review the results from three very large, well-conducted studies over the past several years—the Women's Health Initiative, the Million Women Study, and the Nurses' Health Study—to clarify the relationship between ERT and breast cancer risk.

The Women's Health Initiative study found an increased risk of breast cancer in women using the synthetic estrogen Premarin along with the synthetic progestin Provera (Prempro), but <u>not</u> in women using Premarin alone.[303] The Million Women Study did show an increased risk with ERT (bioidentical and synthetic) and an even higher risk with estrogen plus synthetic progestins.[304] Lastly, the Nurses' Health Study also found an increased risk with long-term (more than 15 years) estrogen replacement, in women who used estrogen alone.[305]

You may recall from the previous section on pellet implants that a few studies (one with 261 women, one with 508 women) have shown no increased risk of breast cancer,[306,307] or risk of recurrence in women who've been treated for breast cancer (123 women)[308] with estradiol pellets, especially if used in combination with testosterone.[309]

As stated earlier, vaginal estrogens, especially estriol, do not increase the risk for breast cancer;[310-314] vaginal estriol also does not increase the risk for recurrence in breast cancer survivors.[315] There is no accumulation of hormones or metabolites with vaginal estrogen or progesterone therapy.[316-318]

The data is irrefutable that **synthetic progestins** (such as Provera®) do significantly increase the risk for breast cancer.

However, bioidentical **progesterone** is a different molecule than synthetic progestins and has a different effect on breast cancer risk.

Progesterone deficiency (in women who don't ovulate or who don't make enough progesterone) has been shown to increase the risk for breast cancer. In one study progesterone deficient women had a 5.4 times increased risk of pre-menopausal breast cancer, and a 10 times increased risk of death from all malignant cancers.[319] Another study evaluated hormone levels in women under age 45 who developed pre-menopausal breast cancer. There was no association between serum SHBG (sex hormone binding globulin), estradiol, testosterone or androstenedione and premenopausal breast cancer risk. The only link was an inverse relationship between risk and luteal phase progesterone levels—women with the highest progesterone levels had the lowest risk.[320] The risk of developing breast cancer seems to be decreased in women with high luteal phase progesterone levels.[321,322]

Breast cancer risk does not increase with the use of **bioidentical progesterone supplementation** (oral micronized progesterone, such as Prometrium,® topical progesterone cream, or intravaginal progesterone).[323-325]

The role of **testosterone** in breast cancer is often confusing, due to the use of synthetic, methyltestosterone versus bioidentical testosterone in many studies. In animal and human studies, testosterone supplementation does not increase breast cancer risk.[326,327]

Testosterone inhibits the growth of breast cancer cells via the androgen receptor.[328-332] Testosterone works by preventing breast cells from dividing and multiplying, and by inducing apoptosis (programmed cell death).[333-337] Adrenal androgens, such as DHEA and androstenedione, and testosterone counteract the way estrogen stimulates the growth of breast cancer cells.[338-340]

Some studies have found that if a woman has androgen-receptor positive breast cancer, her prognosis is better than a woman who doesn't.[341,342] In women with breast cancer treated with anti-estrogens (such as Tamoxifen®), those given androgens have better outcomes.[343,344] Interestingly, synthetic progestins may increase the risk of breast cancer by blocking the androgen receptor and negating the protective effects of testosterone on breast tissue.[345]

Clinical studies have shown that testosterone given as a patch or pellet can prevent breast proliferation and decrease estrogen receptors.[346,347] In addition, women who receive testosterone pellets have been shown to have no increased risk of breast cancer even though they were taking estrogen and synthetic progestins.[348] In one study, testosterone pellets showed no increased risk of recurrence in breast cancer survivors.[349]

Women with a history of breast cancer deserve to be adequately informed about each individual hormone and the risk of cancer recurrence. I recommend breast cancer survivors do not use estradiol replacement, unless safer forms of estrogen (estriol) or bioidentical testosterone pellet implants (often given along with an aromatase inhibitor to prevent conversion to estrogens) have been unsuccessful at alleviating symptoms.

### Lowering your risk for breast cancer

Benjamin Franklin's famous words—*an ounce of prevention is worth a pound of cure*—are certainly applicable to all areas of health. The following recommendations have been shown to lower breast cancer risk:

- **Eat a healthy, Mediterranean-type diet.** This type of diet has been shown to significantly lower breast cancer risk.[350] A Mediterranean diet consists mainly of vegetables, fruit, whole grains, seafood, nuts, and olive oil. The standard American diet (appropriately called the "SAD" diet) consists mainly of meat, fried food, potatoes, pizza, and white flour products—avoid or significantly limit eating a SAD diet.

- **Drink alcohol in moderation or not at all.** One alcoholic drink per day increases breast cancer risk by 10%, and two drinks increase the risk by 20 to 40%.[351]

- **Exercise!** Sustained physical activity for 30-45 minutes, 3 to 7 times per week, has been shown to decrease the risk of breast cancer between 20 and 60%[352,353]

- **If feasible, have children and breast feed at a younger age.** Giving birth before age 25 and having multiple children is known to be breast protective. Most research shows that, regardless of the mother's age, breastfeeding also lowers breast cancer risk.[354,355]

- **Maintain normal weight** — obesity can double or triple your risk for breast cancer.[356-358]

- **Don't smoke.** Cigarettes are known carcinogens for many different types of cancer, including breast cancer.[359] Smoking also dramatically increases free radicals, shortens telomeres, and accelerates aging.

- **Empty your "stress bucket" daily.** Chronic, prolonged stress impairs your cell's ability to repair DNA damage, leading to an increased possibility of defective cell division and cancer formation.[360]

- **Maintain a serum vitamin D level >30 ng/mL, possibly 40-70 ng/mL.** Vitamin D and sunlight exposure are breast cancer protective.[361] If you don't know your vitamin D level, consider supplementing with 1000 IU of vitamin D3 per day; this dosage has been shown to lower overall cancer risk by 60%.[362]

- **Go through a yearly detox program.** Many studies have linked environmental toxins to breast cancer.[363] Yearly detoxification can enable you to minimize exposure and enhance metabolism and excretion of stored toxins. See chapter 9 for detoxification programs and books.

Some nutritional supplements may help lower your risk for breast cancer. They include:

- **Indol-3-carbinol** — 200 to 600 mg per day. Indol-3-carbinol enhances estrogen metabolism and has been shown to lower breast cancer risk.[364]

- **Green tea** contains EGCG (epigallocatechin gallate), which helps block vascular endothelial growth factor (VEGF), preventing formation of blood vessels that feed tumors. Green tea has also been shown to inhibit the growth of cancerous tumors, and increase their death.[365,366] Suggested dosage is 300-1500 mg of green tea capsules per day. For breast cancer prevention, drinking three to five cups of green tea per day is recommended.

- **Melatonin** is a potent antioxidant that inhibits breast cancer cell growth.[367-369] A high percentage of women with breast cancer have low melatonin levels.[370] As previously mentioned, women who work the "graveyard" shift have a higher risk for breast cancer; therefore, avoid working through the night to prevent disruption of this powerful hormone. If you supplement with melatonin, the recommended dosage depends on prevention (3-5 mg before bed) or breast cancer treatment (beneficial dosage may be significantly higher).

- **Fish oil** — Higher omega-3 (fish oil) to omega-6 ratio may reduce the risk of breast cancer.[371,372] Fish oil has been shown to retard the growth of breast cancer in the laboratory, and inhibit breast cancer from developing and spreading in animal studies. Take 1,000 to 6,000 mg EPA and DHA per day.

- **Antioxidants** — especially carotenoids (such as beta-carotene, lycopene, lutein, and zeaxanthin), C, E, selenium, and zinc may lower breast cancer risk, as well as improve telomere length.[373,374]

Understandably, many women are afraid of breast cancer — it is much too common, and is too often fatal. It's essential to remember, however, that women are ten times more likely to die of heart disease than breast cancer. Recall that decreased estrogen and testosterone production are associated with metabolic changes that increase a woman's risk for cardiovascular disease (higher total and LDL cholesterol and triglycerides, and lower HDL cholesterol). In addition, body composition changes that occur with menopause include increased total body fat, especially with accumulation around the waist, and decreased lean body mass. This increased fat to lean body mass and muscle ratio may improve with bioidentical testosterone supplementation. In addition, estrogen replacement can improve cholesterol levels and the health of blood vessels.

Other long-term problems with menopause include bone loss, increased risk of Alzheimer's, thinning skin, urinary frequency, vaginal dryness, tooth and gum disease, weight gain, sleep problems and sexual dysfunction. Considering the fact that bioidentical hormones can help with all of these symptoms and conditions, it's important to weigh your specific risks and benefits when deciding whether to supplement with bioidentical hormones.

## Prostate Cancer

Prostate cancer is, unfortunately, the most common non-skin cancer in the U.S. and the second most common cause of cancer death in men (lung cancer is the first). In 2009, 192,000 men were diagnosed with prostate cancer, with approximately 27,000 deaths. According to the American Cancer Society, one man out of six will develop prostate cancer in his lifetime. Although prostate cancer accounts for 25% of all cancer diagnoses, it causes only 10% of cancer deaths.[375] The good news is that, if diagnosed early, the cure rate for prostate cancer is nearly 100%. To put prostate cancer mortality into perspective, men are more likely to die of heart disease, lung cancer, stroke, emphysema, or pneumonia than from prostate cancer.

As of 2005, more than two million men in the US have, or have had, prostate cancer. The majority of men have localized disease, which means the cancer is only within the prostate gland itself. The risk for prostate cancer increases significantly with age and it is more common in black men. If you have a first-degree relative (father, brother, or son) with prostate cancer, your risk is doubled or tripled.

Current research shows that what men eat significantly affects their risk for prostate cancer. Plant-based foods (fruits and vegetables) contain phytochemicals—carotenoids, flavonoids, phytoestrogens, and isothiocyanates—that have been shown to have anti-carcinogenic properties. Research regarding diet and prostate cancer risk has shown that more than two servings per week of lycopene—found in tomatoes, carrots, watermelon, and papayas—supplies approximately five mg of lycopene daily, which decreases risk.[376,377] More than five servings per week of cruciferous vegetables (e.g., broccoli, cauliflower, mustard greens) also decreases the risk.

Prostate cancer risk is increased with high meat consumption (more than five times per week), especially meat that is cooked at high temperatures. This includes grilled (barbequed) or charred meat, and processed meat such as sausage, bacon, and hot dogs. In addition, high dairy and saturated fat intake also increase the risk.

Obesity is another controllable risk factor for prostate cancer. Obese men have a greater risk of developing more aggressive cancers and of dying from the disease.[378,379] Excess body weight and the link to prostate cancer may be due to elevated insulin, a strong growth factor for cancer. Keeping insulin levels low by limiting simple carbohydrates and sugar, and exercising daily, can lower the risk.

Certain nutrients and supplements, especially vitamin E, selenium, vitamin D, and fish oil, may protect against prostate cancer.[380] The Alpha-Tocopherol Beta-Carotene (ATBC) Cancer Prevention Study revealed that men who take vitamin E have approximately one-third lower risk of developing prostate cancer.[381] Other studies have also reported decreased prostate cancer in men who take vitamin E.[382] Although not all studies are consistent,[383] many studies show that selenium may significantly reduce prostate cancer risk.[384-389] Selenium supplementation (200 to 400 mcg per day) may also slow the progression of prostate cancer.

Prostate cells contain receptors for active vitamin D; these cells respond to vitamin $D_3$ by increasing differentiation, or normal cell maturity, and death of old cells. Vitamin $D_3$ also slows proliferation (cell division) and decreases the spread of cancerous prostate cells.[390] Adequate blood levels of vitamin D significantly reduce the incidence and death for many types of cancer—research has shown that serum vitamin D levels can even predict the likelihood of prostate and other cancers and death in men.[391,392]

### Prostate cancer and hormones

Historically, testosterone was thought to cause prostate cancer. In fact, if your testosterone level is low, your doctor may still believe that giving you bioidentical testosterone will lead to cancer and he or she may caution you against it. It's very important to understand the current research regarding hormones and prostate cancer. A recent meta-analysis of 18 prospective studies examined the relationship between hormones and prostate cancer risk.[393] Overall, data from nearly 4,000 men with prostate cancer and more than 6,000 control subjects (men without prostate cancer) was pooled. No association was seen between the risk of prostate cancer and levels of testosterone, free testosterone, or dihydrotestesterone (DHT). In addition, there was no association with other hormones such as androstenedione, estradiol, or free estradiol.

Curiously, some studies have shown an association between <u>low</u> testosterone levels and prostate cancer.[394,395] In addition, other studies have reported that low testosterone levels are associated with more aggressive prostate cancers (advanced pathological stage and higher Gleason score).[396-400]

A recent pivotal study strongly suggests that testosterone supplementation does not lead to prostate cancer.[401] In this study, 44 men with late-onset hypogonadism (low testosterone) were randomized to receive testosterone or placebo for 6 months. Prostate biopsies were performed prior to the study to rule out prostate cancer and to determine tissue levels of testosterone and DHT (dihydrotestosterone — the potent metabolite of testosterone) within the prostate gland itself. After six months, the 40 men who completed the study underwent repeat biopsies. Although testosterone treatment led to normal serum testosterone levels (median serum testosterone at baseline was 282 ng/dl versus 640 ng/dl after 6 mos), no significant changes were reported regarding levels of testosterone or DHT in the prostate, and no changes associated with prostate cancer were found.

### *Prostate cancer prevention*

As you now know, one man in six will develop prostate cancer in his lifetime, and the risk increases with age. Most men with prostate cancer do not die from the disease. Prostate cancer may be preventable by following these guidelines:

- Eat more than two servings of lycopene rich foods per week (e.g., tomatoes, carrots, watermelon, and papaya).
- Include at least five servings of cruciferous vegetables (broccoli, cauliflower, mustard greens, cabbage) in your diet every week.
- Keep meat consumption to a minimum (especially charred, barbequed, or processed meat).
- Avoid excess dairy products and saturated fat.
- If you're overweight or obese, commit to a weight-loss plan. Men who gain a significant amount of weight after age 21 have a higher risk for prostate cancer.[402]
- Supplement with vitamins E and D, selenium, and fish oil.

# Chapter 9: Optimal Aging Questionnaire & Resources

Now that you're armed with knowledge about how aging happens, what hormones do, symptoms of imbalance, optimal aging tests, and *"The 8 Steps to Achieving HormoneSynergy,"* I hope you're ready to translate information into action. The following questionnaire will help you identify how well you're doing and where you need help. Place a check in the boxes where you already practice optimal aging behaviors. The unchecked boxes will help you identify where you need improvement. The "Tools" section provides ideas and resources for improving your health and slowing or reversing the aging process.

## *HormoneSynergy Optimal Aging Questionnaire*

☐ **1. I have an internal locus of control about my health.**
- "Locus of control" refers to your perception about the main causes of events in your life. In this case, it means that <u>you are responsible for your health</u>. Having an "internal locus of control" means that nobody—not your doctor, spouse, boss, fast food restaurants, the media, lack of time, your insurance company, or the medical establishment—defines or limits your health. Longevity is at least 66% lifestyle choices. With an internal locus of control, you have the power to seek out information (such as this book) and live a healthy, vibrant life.

☐ **2. Currently, I am in excellent health.**
- I have no major diseases, health problems, or chronic symptoms.

- My energy level, on a scale of 1 to 10, is usually ≥ 8 on most days.
- I experience joy on a daily basis and feel happy and free.

☐ **3. I manage stress well, and I "empty my stress bucket" every day.**

☐ **4. My diet is excellent.**
- I focus on what I should eat every day, including:
  - Minimum—5 to 7 servings of vegetables and fruit per day (organic as much as possible)
  - Protein—15 to 30 grams, 3 x day including beans nuts, free-range, lean meat, fish (wild, not farm raised), eggs, and protein powders (whey, soy, rice).
- I avoid most processed foods and refined sugar.
- I eat healthy fats (fish, avocadoes, nuts, olive oil, organic butter) and no hydrogenated oil or trans fat (fried food, packaged baked goods, shortening, margarine).
- I drink two liters of clean, filtered water per day. Teas, especially green and herbal, count as water intake.
- I drink no or a minimal amount of alcohol—ideally, no more than one drink per day.

☐ **5. I exercise, 30-60 minutes, 5-7 x week.**
- I exercise at the intensity needed for cardiovascular fitness (minimum of 30-45 minutes at 60-80% of my maximum heart rate).

☐ **6. I keep my brain healthy by:**
- Learning new things and remaining curious
- Keeping  physically active
- Lowering stress
- Taking vitamin D and fish oil
- Sleeping well and enough
- Making sure my hormones are balanced

☐ **7. I sleep well and enough.**
- 7-9 hours per night
- I wake feeling refreshed

☐ **8. My weight is healthy.**
- Healthy weight is defined by body mass index or BMI. Healthy BMI is 18.5 to 24.9; BMI of 25-29.9 is overweight; BMI >30 is obese; BMI >40 is extreme or morbid obesity. See www.nhlbisupport.com/bmi/ to determine your BMI.

☐ **9. My toxicity level is low and I take part in a yearly detox program.**

☐ **10. I take optimal aging supplements to support every cell in my body. (see Tools for recommendations.)**

☐ **11. My hormones are balanced and I re-evaluate them every year.**

### *Tools*

This questionnaire should help you identify areas where you need to focus on your health. Consider hiring professionals to help you achieve your goals—there is no investment as important as your health. If you are not vibrant and healthy, and you're spending money on "things" to make you feel better, you may want to re-evaluate your priorities. Hiring experts who can help you achieve your health goals, is the most important thing you can do for yourself—you deserve to be vibrant and healthy! Examples of consultants you can hire include:

- Physician who specializes in optimal aging
- Certified Life Coach
- Therapist or spiritual director
- Nutritionist
- Personal meal planner or chef
- Personal trainer

1. **Internal locus of control.** If you need help creating vibrant health and the life of your dreams, an excellent book to start with is Will Bowen's *Complaint Free World*. If you do not want to maintain an internal locus of control, consider putting money aside for nursing home and medication costs (since it's unlikely that Medicare or your insurance company will cover all the care you'll need). Consider this—the average Medicare

patient uses more than 4 drugs per day, and 25% use 6 or more. If this is tolerable to you, continue with conventional, disease-based care. If not, recognize that you are responsible for your health and take charge of it today.

2. **Excellent health.** If you're not currently in excellent health, please invest in achieving it. Nothing feels as good as being healthy and vibrant!

3. **Stress.** Stress is not what happens to you, it's how you respond to what happens to you. Chronic stress can lead to weight gain, memory problems, brain degeneration, depression, and anxiety. It can also cause immune system dysfunction including an increased risk for developing frequent infections, autoimmune diseases, and cancer. Learning to "turn off" the stress response in times where it's not needed is a valuable tool. In addition, practicing meditation or yoga, keeping a gratitude journal, or listening to visualization or hypnosis CDs daily can "empty your stress bucket" and prevent it from overflowing.

4. **Diet.** Prioritize your diet and focus on what you need to eat for proper cellular function every day. Food is information for your genes and you literally become what you eat. Stop and think about this. Ask yourself if you've eaten your recommended servings of fruit and vegetables and protein every day. Keep a diet diary to be honest about what and why you eat. If you eat for emotional reasons, identify this and get help changing it—for your health's sake, you must learn to "eat to live" not "live to eat."

5. **Exercise.** Just do it! Consider using a pedometer or bodybugg® to provide feedback and keep you accountable—goal is at least 10,000 steps per day on the pedometer; a bodybugg keeps track of the calories you burn. Do not turn on the TV until you've completed your exercise goal. To achieve cardiovascular fitness, you need to exercise between 60 and 80 percent of your maximum heart rate, for a minimum of 30 minutes, 5 times per week. To find your maximum heart rate, subtract your age from 220; multiply by 0.6 to get 60%, and 0.8 to get 80%. If you have a motivation problem, consider joining a gym,

committing to exercise with a friend, or hiring a personal trainer or Life Coach.

6. **Brain health.** Stimulate your brain through variety and curiosity. Learn new things, do puzzles such as Sudoku or crosswords, or engage in social interaction such as ballroom dancing. The brain chemical BDNF (brain derived neurotrophic factor) is critical for maintaining connections between neurons and creating new ones, and for supporting positive mood.[403] Exercise, learning, stress reduction, fish oil, vitamin D, estradiol, and testosterone can all enhance brain health or increase BDNF.[404-412]

7. **Sleep.** If you're not sleeping well or enough, recognize this as a health problem and seek help. Sleep deprivation has been linked to brain problems such as depression, decreased concentration, and poor memory. In addition, lack of sleep can cause weakened immunity, poor wound healing, and an increased risk for heart disease, diabetes, and weight gain. If your sleep problem is severe, or if you snore or your bed partner says you have lapses in breathing, see a sleep medicine specialist.

8. **Healthy weight.** If you know you're overweight, you owe it to yourself to stop hiding. Get real by getting on the scale and determining your BMI. You can also determine your fat and muscle percentage (more important than overall weight) by using a bioelectrical impedance analysis (BIA). After getting real, please stop beating yourself up about your weight — forgive yourself and find help. Stop dieting and commit to permanent weight loss, meaning you must change your eating, moving, and thinking. There are no shortcuts.

9. **Toxicity.** Unfortunately, we are all toxic. Eliminating what you can by avoiding plastics and eating organic produce and free-range meat is essential to limiting your exposure. In addition, go through a detox program every year to support liver function, eliminate stored toxins, and enhance your health and longevity.

10. **Supplements.** Supplements should be used in addition to, not in place of, adhering to the previous steps. Make sure the supplements you're taking are pharmaceutical quality (not

over-the-counter "food grade') and are certified for good manufacturing practices (GMP). Recommended supplements to support healthy aging include:

- Multi vitamin and mineral
- Antioxidants
- CoQ10
- Fish oil
- Vitamin D3
- Resveratrol

11. **Hormone balance.** Most hormones decline with age, and aging accelerates as hormone levels decline. Hormones are vital for repair of tissues and regulating body functions. There is certainly much controversy about whether or not it's appropriate to restore hormones to youthful levels as people age. Most important is to optimize your body's own hormone production by following the previous 10 steps. If you choose to use hormone replacement, please become informed about risks, benefits, and options.

# *Resources*

**Organizations who support Optimal Aging**

**The Methuselah Foundation:** <u>www.mfoundation.org</u>
> The Methuselah Foundation is a nonprofit medical charity dedicated to extending healthy human life. The foundation supports a variety of strategies that accelerate progress toward a comprehensive cure for age-related disease, disability, and suffering.

**The Life Extension Foundation:** <u>www.lef.org</u>
> The Life Extension Foundation is a nonprofit organization whose long-range goal is the extension of the healthy human lifespan. The Life Extension Foundation has well-referenced articles and information about anti-aging topics on its website. The organization also sells an extensive list of quality supplements. Membership includes a subscription to the monthly *Life Extension* magazine, access to health advisors about nutrition, and discounted supplements and lab work.

**The International Hormone Society:**
<u>www.intlhormonesociety.org</u>
> The International Hormone Society has two goals: First is to make the public aware of the importance and availability of doctors specializing in the medical science of hormone deficiencies or excesses and in the medicine of aging. The second goal is to work within the medical community to bring the "medicine of aging" to a more prominent level among the various medical specialties. The IHS is a reliable source for accurate information regarding hormones and optimal aging.

**The American Academy for Anti-Aging Medicine:**
<u>www.worldhealth.net</u>
> The American Academy of Anti-Aging Medicine (A4M) is a non-profit organization comprised of more than 22,000 physicians, health practitioners, scientists, governmental officials, and members of the general public, representing more than 105 nations. The A4M educates the health care community about research and treatment modalities designed to prolong human lifespan.

## To learn more about Bioidentical Hormones

### HormoneSynergy: www.hormonesynergy.com

HormoneSynergy's mission is to educate and inspire people to achieve hormone balance and optimal health. The website contains an extensive list of references on BHRT and research on subcutaneous pellet implants. Interviews, presentations, videos, and downloadable CDs on topics related to optimal aging and health are also available.

### Women In Balance: www.womeninbalance.org

Women In Balance provides information about hormones, educational conferences, research, and resources to enable women to take charge of their hormone health.

### Rebecca Glaser, MD: www.hormonebalance.org

Dr. Glaser's website is a treasure of information on hormones, including research, resources, and educational handouts and presentations. As a former breast cancer surgeon, Dr. Glaser places special emphasis on hormones and breast cancer risk and is currently investigating testosterone pellets, their ability to alleviate menopausal symptoms, and breast cancer risk.

## Tools for Stress Reduction:

### Daniel Soule, CHt, Certified Professional Coach: www.hormonesynergy.com

Download Daniel's free guided visualization, self-hypnosis session, *"Emptying Your Stress Bucket."*

### Eckhart Tolle: www.eckharttolle.com

Eckhart Tolle's books, especially *The Power of Now* and *Stillness Speaks*, contain teachings that enable you to return to the present moment and to find the "off switch" for your mind.

### Will Bowen: www.acomplaintfreeworld.org

A Complaint Free World, Inc. is a non-profit, non-religious organization that provides Complaint Free purple bracelets and other materials to help people focus on the positive aspects of their lives, and manifest the life they want. Consider taking the "Complaint Free" challenge of going 21 days without complaining to transform your relationships and your life.

## Sleep Help

### Daniel Soule, CHt, Certified Professional Coach:
### www.souletosoul.com

Daniel's website provides information about life coaching and hypnosis to help with sleep problems, as well as weight issues, smoking, or significant stress. You'll also find hypnosis CDs to help your subconscious mind remember how to sleep on the HormoneSynergy website: www.hormonesynergy.com.

### Wendi Friesen, CHt: www.wendi.com

Wendi's website contains information about hypnosis and CDs to help with dozens of problems including insomnia. There are several free sessions to try and videos about changing habits, beliefs, and behaviors.

### Alpha-Stim®: www.alpha-stim.com

The Alpha-Stim is a medical device that applies low-dose electrical treatment to the brain. Extensive research on the device has shown it to be very safe and effective and it is FDA-approved. The Alpha-Stim is a valuable, non-drug option for people who struggle with sleep problems, pain, depression, or anxiety.

## Detoxification Products

7 Day Detox Miracle, Peter Bennett, ND & Stephen Barrie, ND. New York: Three Rivers Press, 2001.

Drs. Bennet and Barrie have provided readers with a comprehensive manual about the purpose and benefits of detoxification, and how to undergo a safe, effective detox program.

### UltraClear Plus, available from Metagenics:
### www.metagenics.com

UltraClear Plus is a medical food designed to support detoxification pathways in the liver. The clinically researched program includes following a hypoallergenic, anti-inflammatory diet while using UltraClear Plus for 21 to 28 days.

### MediClear Plus, available from Thorne Research, Inc:
### www.thorne.com

MediClear Plus is a rice protein-based product containing vitamins, minerals, amino acids, botanicals, probiotics, and other nutrients to enhance detoxification and lower inflammation.

## Liver C, available from Mountain Peak Nutritionals: www.mpn8.com

Liver C contains botanicals, mushrooms, vitamins, and minerals designed to optimize liver function. Milk thistle has been shown to regenerate liver cells, alpha-lipoic acid raises glutathione levels, and turmeric protects the liver and lowers inflammation.

# Supplements

## HormoneSynergy: www.hormonesynergy.com

My website includes a comprehensive on-line store featuring products to support optimal aging, women's and men's health, detoxification, and adrenal, immune, cardiovascular, brain, and gastrointestinal function. I've personally researched all products and have used them with exceptional results in my clinical practice.

## Douglas Laboratories: www.douglaslabs.com

Douglas Labs surpasses GMP standards, including GMP certification, by constantly monitoring quality via their certified in-house laboratories. They ensure raw materials used in supplements are tested for microbes and contaminants, and they analyze all products for potency.

## Metagenics: www.metagenics.com

Metagenics is a pioneer in supplement manufacturing since they have an on-sight, medically supervised functional medicine institute where they perform clinical trials on their products. In addition to GMP, TGA, and NSF certification, safety review of all ingredients, and performing clinical trials, Metagenics has designed a therapeutic lifestyle program (First Line Therapy®) that enables people to implement healthy diet, detoxification, exercise, and stress management habits to improve health and longevity.

**Thorne Research, Inc:** www.thorne.com

Thorne products are formulated to be hypoallergenic and are manufactured in powders or capsules free of additives, flowing agents, or binders. Thorne is GMP and TGA certified and performs in-house analysis of products for quality assurance. Thorne also publishes the *Alternative Medicine Review*, a peer-reviewed journal designed to disseminate information on the practical use of alternative and complementary therapies.

**Mountain Peak Nutritionals:** www.mpn8.com

Mountain Peak Nutritionals was founded by a well-respected, experienced naturopathic physician, Jim Massey, ND, to provide high-quality, condition specific formulas that are manufactured in compliance with good manufacturing practices (GMP).

**Nordic Naturals**: www.nordicnaturals.com

An excellent source for high-potency, pure fish oil.

## Compounding Pharmacies & Resources

**Professional Compounding Centers of America:** www.pccarx.com

The PCCA provides continuing education and training for pharmacists and physicians, as well as a source of FDA-approved compounding ingredients subjected to rigorous quality assurance standards.

**Pharmacy Compounding Accreditation Board (PCAB):**
www.pcab.org

PCAB-accredited pharmacies have demonstrated superior quality and safety in compounding practices. The steps to becoming accredited are stringent and expensive, however PCAB certification enables consumers to trust that certified pharmacies produce reliable, safe products.

**McGuff Compounding Pharmacy:** www.mcguffpharmacy.com

McGuff Pharmacy is PCAB accredited and ISO certified, and is one of the most respected compounding pharmacies in the industry. The pharmacists at McGuff are very knowledgeable and willing to discuss hormones and compounding with patients and physicians.

## Laboratories

There are many laboratories providing standard blood tests. Following are labs that offer optimal aging testing.

**Genova Diagnostics: www.genovadiagnostics.com**

Genova Diagnostics offers functional medicine testing in most areas of health and SNP testing (single nucleotide polymorphisms—genetic variations in genes) to determine predispositions for certain diseases and conditions. Genova also performs phase I and II liver function testing, and toxic metal (aluminum, arsenic, cadmium, lead, and mercury) testing.

**SpectraCell Laboratories, Inc: www.spectracell.com**

SpectraCell offers micronutrient and advanced lipoprotein particle testing (to assess cardiovascular risk). They also perform telomere testing (to measure cellular age) at an affordable price.

**ZRT Laboratory: www.zrtlab.com**

ZRT Laboratory offers convenient salivary and blood spot testing to detect hormone imbalances, cardio metabolic risk, and vitamin D deficiency.

# REFERENCES

[1] Okinawa Centenarian Study: www.okicent.org/study.html

[2] Vermeulen A, Kaufman J, Goemaere S, VanPottelberg I. Estradiol in elderly men. *The Aging Male* 2002; 5(2):98-102.

[3] Maggio M, Lauretani F, Ceda G, et al. Estradiol and metabolic syndrome in older Italian men: the InCHIANTI study. *J Andrology*. 2010;31(2):155-62.

[4] Behl C, Skutella T, Lezoualch F, et al. Neuroprotection against oxidative stress by estrogens: structure-activity relationship. *Mol Pharmacol* 1997;51:535-541.

[5] Singer CA, Figueroa-Masot XA, Batchelor RH, Dorsa DM. The mitogen-activated protein kinase pathway mediates estrogen neuroprotection after glutamate toxicity in primary cortical neurons. *J Neuroscience* 1999;19:2455-2463.

[6] Zandi P, Carlson M, Plassman B, et al. Hormone replacement therapy and incidence of Alzheimer disease in older women: the cache county study. *JAMA* 2002;288:2123-2129.

[7] Zonderman A. Predicting Alzheimer's disease in the Baltimore Longitudinal Study of Aging. *J Geriatr Psychiatry Neurol* 2005;18(4):192-5.

[8] Cohen L, Soares C, Poitra, et al. Short-term use of estradiol for depression in perimenopausal and postmenopausal women: a preliminary report. *Am J Psychiatry* 2003 Aug;160(8):1519-22.

[9] Kaur K, Cooper MS, Arlt W, et al. Inactivating progesterone metabolism in human osteoblasts. *Endocrine Abstracts* 2004;7:10.

[10] Tremollieres F, Strong D, Baylink D, et al. Progesterone and promegestone stimulate human bone cell proliferation and insulin-like growth factor-2 production. *Acta Endocrinologica* (Copenh)1992;126(4)329-337.

[11] Barud W, Piotrowska-Swirszcz A, Ostrowski S, et al. Association of obesity and insulin resistance with serum testosterone, sex hormone binding globulin and estradiol in older males. *Pol Merkur Lekarski*. 2005 Nov:19(113):634-7.

[12] Ding EL, Song Y, Malik VS, Liu S. Sex differences of exogenous sex hormones and risk of type II diabetes. *JAMA*. 2006 295(11):1288-99.

[13] Pitteloud N, Mootha V, Dwyer A, et al. Relationship between testosterone levels, insulin sensitivity, and mitochondrial function in men. *Diabetes Care*. 2005 28(7):1636-1642.

[14] Tibblin G, Adlerberth A, Lindstedt G, et al. The pituitary-gonadal axis and health in elderly men: a study of men born in 1913. *Diabetes.* 1996 Nov;45(11):1605-9.

[15] Rice D, Brannigan RE, Campbell RK, et al. Men's health, low testosterone, and diabetes: individualized treatment and a multidisciplinary approach. *Diabetes Educ.* 2008;Supl 5:97S-112S.

[16] Simon D, Charles M, Nahoul K, et al. Association between plasma total testosterone and cardiovascular risk factors in healthy adult men: The Telecom Study. *J Clin Endocrin Metab.* 1997 82(2): 682-5.

[17] Fogari R, Zoppi A, Preti P, et al. Sexual activity and plasma testosterone levels in hypertensive males. *Am J Hypertension.* 2002; 15:217–221.

[18] Phillips GB, Jing TY, Resnick LM, et al. Sex hormones and hemostatic risk factors for coronary heart disease in men with hypertension. *J Hypertension.* 1993; 11:699–702.

[19] Khaw KT, Barrett-Connor E. Blood pressure and endogenous testosterone in men: an inverse relationship. *J Hypertension.* 1998; 6:329–332.

[20]Webb C, McNeill J, Hayward C. Effects of testosterone on coronary vasomotor regulation in men with coronary heart disease. *Circulation.* 1999;100:1690-1696.

[21] Rubinow DR, Schmidt, PJ. Androgens, brain, and behavior. *Am J Psychiatry.* 1996; 153:974-984.

[22] Moffatt SD, Zonderman AB, Metter EF, et al. Free testosterone and risk for Alzheimer disease in older men. *Neurology.* 2004;62:188-93.

[23] Hogervorst E, Bandelow S, Combrinck M, et al. Low free testosterone is an independent risk factor for Alzheimer's disease. *Exp Gerontol.* 2004;39(11-12):1633-9.

[24] Pike CJ, Rosario ER, Nguyen TV. Androgens, aging, and Alzheimer's disease. *Endocrine.* 2006;29(2):233-41.

[25] Hull E, Muschamp J, Sato S. Dopamine and serotonin: influences on male sexual behavior. *Physiol Behav.* 2004;83:291-307.

[26]Hull E, Du J, Lorrain D, et al. Testosterone, preoptic dopamine, and copulation in male rats. *Brain Res Bulletin.* 1997; 44(4):327-333.

[27] Okun MS, McDonald WM, DeLong MR. Refractory nonmotor symptoms in male patients with Parkinson disease due to testosterone deficiency: a common unrecognized comorbidity. *Arch Neurol.* 2002; 59(5):807-11.

[28] Ready RE. Testosterone deficiency and apathy in Parkinson's disease: a pilot study. *J Neurol Neurosurg Psychiatry.* 2004;75(9):1323-6.

[29] Okun MS. Beneficial effects of testosterone replacement for the nonmotor symptoms of Parkinson disease. *Arch Neurol.* 2002;59(11)1750-3.

[30] Glei DA, Goldman N. Dehydroepiandrosterone sulfate (DHEAS) and risk for mortality among older Taiwanese. *Ann Epidemiol.* 2006;16(7):510-5.

[31] Mazat L, Lafont S, Berr C, et al. Prospective measurements of dehydroepiandrosterone sulfate in a cohort of elderly subjects: relationship to gender, subjective health, smoking habits, and 10-year mortality. *PNAS.* 2001;98(14):8145-50.

[32] Thomas N, Morris HA, Scopacasa F, et al. Relationships between age, dehydroepiandrosterone sulphate and plasma glucose in healthy men. *Age Ageing* 1999;28(2):217-20.

[33] Paolisso G, Ammendola S, Rotondi M, et al. Insulin resistance and advancing age: what role for dehydroepiandrosterone sulfate? *Metabolism.* 1997 Nov;46(11):1281-6.

[34] Barry NN, McGuire JL, van Vollenhoven RF. Dehydroepiandrosterone in systemic lupus erythematosus: relationship between dosage, serum levels, and clinical response. *J Rheumatol* 1998;25:2352-2356.

[35] Deighton CM, Watson MJ, Walker DJ. Sex hormones in postmenopausal HLA-identical rheumatoid arthritis discordant sibling pairs. *J Rheumatol.* 1992, 19:1663-1667.

[36] Luppi C, Fioravanti M, Bertolini B, et al. Growth factors decrease in subjects with mild to moderate Alzheimer's disease (AD): potential correction with dehydroepiandrosterone-sulphate (DHEA-S). *Arch Gerontol Geriatr.* 2009;49 Suppl 1:173-84.

[37] Bauer ME. Chronic stress and immunosenescence: a review. *Neuroimmunomodulation.* 2008;15(4-6):241-50.

[38] Gouin JP, Hantsoo L, Kiecolt-Glaser JK. Immune dysregulation and chronic stress among older adults: a review. *Neuroimmunomodulation.* 2008;15(4-6):251-9.

[39] Bauer ME, Jeckel CM, Luz C. The role of stress factors during aging of the immune system. *Ann N Y Acad Sci.* 2009;1153:139-52.

[40] Burford TW, Willoughby DS. Impact of DHEA(S) and cortisol on immune function in aging: a brief review. *Appl Physiol Nutr Metab.* 2008;33(3):429-33.

[41] Parducz A, Hajszan T, Maclusky NJ, et al. Synaptic remodeling induced by gonadal hormones: neuronal plasticity as a mediator of neuroendocrine and behavioral responses to steroids. *Neuroscience.* 2006;138(3):977-85.

[42] Bologa L, Sharma J, Roberts E. Dehydroepiandrosterone and its sulfated derivative reduce neuronal death and enhance astrocytic differentiation in brain cell cultures. *J Neurosci Res.* 1987;17(3):225-34.

[43] Cardounel A, Regelson W, Kalimi M. Dehydroepiandrosterone protects hippocampal neurons against neurotoxin-induced cell death: mechanism of action. *Proc Soc Exp Biol Med.* 1999, 222:145-149.

[44] Wolkowitz OM, Reus VI, Keebler A, et al. Double-blind treatment of major depression with dehydroepiandrosterone. *Am J Psychiatry.* 1999, 156:646-649.

[45] Bloch M, Schmidt PJ, Danaceau MA, et al. Dehydroepiandrosterone treatment of midlife dysthymia. *Biol Psychiatry.* 1999, 45:1533-1541.

[46] Kirkegaard C, Faber J. The role of thyroid hormones in depression. *Eur J Endocrinol.* 1998;138(1):1–9.

[47] Dratman M, Gordon J. Thyroid hormones as neurotransmitters. *Thyroid.* 1996;6(6):639–47.

[48] CDC: National Diabetes Fact Sheet, 2007.

[49] Hu F, Manson J, Stampfer M, et al. Diet, Lifestyle, and the risk of type 2 diabetes mellitus in women. *N Engl J Med.* 2001.345(11):790-7.

[50] Bao BY, Yao J, Lee YF. 1-alpha,25-dihydroxyvitamin D3 suppresses interleukin-8-mediatd prostate cancer cell angiogenesis. *Carcinogenesis.* 2006 Sep;27(9):1883-93.

[51] Trump DL, Deeb KK, Johnson CS. Vitamin D: considerations in the continued development as an agent for cancer prevention and therapy. *Cancer J.* 2010;16(1):1-9.

[52] Lappe JM, Travers-Gustafson D, Davies KM, et al. Vitamin D and calcium supplementation reduces cancer risk: results of a randomized trial. *Am J Clin Nutr.* 2007;85(6):1586-91.

[53] Richards J, Valdes A, Gardner J, et al. Higher serum vitamin D concentrations are associated with longer leukocyte telomere length in women. *Am J Clin Nutr.* 2007;86(5):1420-1425.

[54] Gorbach S. Estrogens, breast cancer, and intestinal flora. Rev Infect Dis. 1984;6(suppl 1):S85-S90.

[55] Carwile J, Luu H, Bassett L, et al. Polycarbonate bottle use and urinary bisphenol A concentrations. *Environmental Health Perspectives.* 2009;117(9):1368-1372.

[56] Doll M. The premenstrual syndrome: effectiveness of Vitex agnus castus. [Article in German]. *Med Monatsschr Pharm.* 2009;32(5):186-91.

[57] Schellenberg R. Treatment for the premenstrual syndrome with agnus castus fruit extract: prospective, randomized, placebo controlled study. *BMJ.* 2001;322(7270):134-7.

[58] Nelson LR, Bulun SE. Estrogen production and action. *J Am Acad Dermatol.* 2001;43(3 Suppl):S116-24.

[59] Simpson ER. Sources of estrogen and their importance. *J Steroid Biochem Mol Biol.* 2003;86(3-5):225-30.

[60] Zumoff B, Stain G, Miller L, et al. Twenty-four-hour mean plasma testosterone concentration declines with age in normal premenopausal women. *J Clin Endocrinol Metab.* 1995; 80(4):1429-40.

[61] Davison SL, Bell R, Donath S, et al. Androgen levels in adult females: changes with age, menopause, and oophorectomy. *J Clin Endocrinol Metab.* 2005;90:3847-3853.

[62] van Geel T, Geusens P, Winkens B, et al. Measures of bioavailable serum testosterone and estradiol and their relationships with muscle mass, muscle strength and bone mineral density in postmenopausal women: a cross-sectional study. *European J Endocrinol.* 2009;160:681.

[63] Corlett GL, Pugh PJ, Kapoor D, et al. Testosterone increases interleukin 10, an anti-inflammatory cytokine, in whole blood from hypogonadal men. Presented at the British Endocrine Societies Joint Meeting. *Endocrine Abstracts.* 2002;3P252.

[64] Malkin C, Pugh P, Jones R, et al. The effect of testosterone replacement on endogenous inflammatory cytokines and lipid profiles in hypogonadal men. *Clin Endocrinol Metab.* 2004;89(7):3313-18.

[65] Travison T, Araujo A, O'Donnell B, et al. A population-level decline in serum testosterone levels in American men. *J Clin Endorcrinol Metab.* 2006; 92(1):16-202.

[66] Mulligan T, Frick MF, Zuraw QC, et al. Prevalence of hypogonadism in males aged at least 45 years: the HIM study. *Int J Clin Pract.* 2006;60(7):762-769.

[67] Harman SM, Metter EJ, Tobin JD, Pearson J, Blackman MR. Longitudinal effects of aging on serum total and free testosterone levels in healthy men. Baltimore Longitudinal Study of Aging. *J Clin Endocrinol Metab.* 2001;86(2):724-731.

[68] Shabsigh R. Testosterone therapy in erectile dysfunction and hypogonadism. *J Sex Med.* 2005;2(6):785-92.

[69] Blute M, Hakimian P, Kashanian J, et al. Erectile dysfunction and testosterone deficiency. *Front Horm Res.* 2009;37:108-22.

[70] Buvat J, Bou Jaoude G. Significance of hypogonadism in erectile dysfunction. *World J Urol.* 2006;24(6):657-67.

[71] Osuna JA, Bomez-Perez R, Arata-Bellarbarba G, et al. Relationship between BMI, total testosterone, sex hormone-binding globulin, leptin, insulin and insulin resistance in obese men. *Arch Androl.* 2006;52(5):355-61.

[72] Barret-Connor EL. Testosterone and risk factors for cardiovascular disease in men. *Diabetes Metab.* 1995;21:156-161.

[73] Kiel DP, Baron CA, Plymate SR. Sex hormones and lipoproteins in men. *Am J Med.* 1989; 87: 35-39.

[74] Hergenc, G, Schulte, H, Assmann, G, et al. Associations of obesity markers, insulin, and sex hormones with HDL-cholesterol levels in Turkish and German individuals. *Atherosclerosis.* 1999;145: 147-156.

[75] Simon D, Charles MA, Nahoul K, et al. Association between plasma total testosterone and cardiovascular risk factors in healthy adult men: The Telecom Study. J *Clin Endocrinol Metab.* 1997;82:682-685.

[76] Svartberg J, von Muhlen D, Schirmer H, et al. Associations of endogenous testosterone with blood pressure and left ventricular mass in men. The Tromso Study. *Eur J Endocrinol.* 2004;150(1):65-71.

[77] Malkin CJ, Pugh PJ, Jones TH, et al. Testosterone for secondary prevention in men with ischaemic heart disease? *Q J Med.* 2003;96:521-529.

[78] Irwin M, Daniels M, Risch S, et al. Plasma cortisol and natural killer cell activity during bereavement. *Biol Psychiatry.* 1988;24:173-178.

[79] Sieber W, Rodin J, Larson L, et al. Modulation of human natural killer cell activity by exposure to uncontrollable stress. *Brain Behav Immun.* 1992;6(2):141-156.

[80] Sergerstrom S, Miller G. Psychological stress and the human immune system: a meta-analytic study of 30 years of inquiry. *Psycological Bulletin.* 2004;130(4):601-30.

[81] Weiss S. Neurobiological alterations associated with traumatic stress. *Perspectives in Psychiatric Care.* 2007; 43:114-122.

[82] Wurtman J, Wurtman R, Growdon J, et al. Carbohydrate cravings in obese people: suppression by treatments affecting serotoninergic transmission. *Int J Eating Disorders.* 1981;1(1):2-15.

[83] Wallin M, Rissanen A. Food and mood: relationship between food, serotonin and affective disorders. *Acta Psychiatrica Scandinavica.* 1994;89(s377):36-40.

[84] Cangiano C, Laviano A, Del Ben M, et al. Effects of oral 5-hydroxytryptophan on energy intake and macronutrient selection in non-insulin dependent diabetic patients. *Int J Obes Relat Metab Disord.* 1998;22(7):648-54.

[85] Rizza RA, Mandarino LJ, Gerich JE. Cortisol-induced insulin resistance in man: impaired suppression of glucose production and stimulation of glucose utilization due to a postreceptor detect of insulin action. *J Clin Endocrinol Metab.* 1982;54(1):131-138.

[86] Wang M. The role of glucocorticoid action in the pathophysiology of the metabolic syndrome. *Nutr Metab (Lond).* 2005;2(1):3.

[87] Epel E, McEwen B, Seeman T, et al. Stress and body shape: stress-induced cortisol secretion is consistently greater among women with central fat. *Psychosomatic Medicine.* 2000;62(5):623-632.

[88] Tomlinson JW, Stewart PM. The functional consequences of 11 B-hydroxysteroid dehydrogenase expression in adipose tissue. *Hormone Metabolic Research.* 2001;34(11-12):746-751.

[89] Epel E, Lapidus R, McEwen B, et al. Stress may add bite to appetite in women: a laboratory study of stress-induced cortisol and eating behavior. *Psychoneuroendocrinology.* 2001;26(1):37-49.

[90] Dinan T. Glucocorticoids and the genesis of depressive illness: a psychobiological model. *Br J Psychiatry.* 1994;164(3):365-371.

[91] Christensen L, Pettijohn L. Mood and carbohydrate cravings. *Appetite.* 2001;36(2):137-145.

[92] Rubello D, Sonino N, Casara D, et al. Acute and chronic effects of high glucocorticoid levels on hypothalamic-pituitary-thyroid axis in man. *J Endocrinol Invest.* 1992;15(6):437-441.

[93] Bános C, Takó J, Salamon F, et al. Effect of ACTH-stimulated glucocorticoid hypersecretion on the serum concentrations of thyroxine-binding globulin, thyroxine, triiodothyronine, reverse triiodothyronine and on the TSH-response to TRH. *Acta Med Acad Scie Hung.* 1979;36(4):381-394.

[94] Kuo L, Kitlinska J, Tilan J, et al. Neuropeptide Y acts directly in the periphery on fat tissue and mediates stress-induced obesity and metabolic syndrome. *Nat Med.* 2007(13):803-811.

[95] Cavagnini F, Croci M, Putignano P, et al. Glucocorticoids and neuroendocrine function. *Int J Obesity.* 2000;24(Suppl 2):S77-S79.

[96] Dratman M, Gordon J. Thyroid hormones as neurotransmitters. *Thyroid.* 1996;6(6):639–47.

[97] Kirkegaard C, Faber J. The role of thyroid hormones in depression. *Eur J Endocrinol* 1998;138(1):1–9.

[98] For more information, see the AACE website: www.aace.com/public/awareness/tam/2003/explanation.php

[99] Tornhage CJ. Salivary cortisol for assessment of hypothalamic-pituitary-adrenal axis function. *Neuroimmunomodulation.* 2009;16(5):284-9.

[100] Gozansky WS, Lynn JS, Laudenslager ML, et al. Salivary cortisol determined by enzyme immunoassay is preferable to serum total cortisol for assessment of dynamic hypothalamic-pituitary-adrenal axis activity. *Clin Endocrinol (Oxf).* 2005;63(3):336-41.

[101] Papanicolaou D, Mullen N, Kyrou I, et al. Nighttime salivary cortisol: a useful test for the diagnosis of cushing's syndrome. *J Clin Endocrinol Metab.* 2002;87(10):4515-4521.

[102] Shinkai S, Watanabe S, Kurokawa Y, et al. Salivary cortisol for monitoring circadian rhythm variation in adrenal activity during shiftwork. *Int Arch Occup Environ Health.* 1993;64(7):499-502.

[103] Rubinstein J, Meyer D, Evans J. Executive Control of Cognitive Process in Task Switching. *J Exp Psychol Hum Percept Perform.* 2001;27(4):763-767.

[104] Ophir E, Nass C, Wagner A. Cognitive control in media multitaskers. *PNAS*. 2009;106:15583-15587.

[105] The case for doing one thing at a time. Sunday, Jan 08, 2006. www.time.com/time/magazine/article/0,9171,1147162,00.html

[106] Berk LS, Tan SA, Fry WF, et al. Neuroendocrine and stress hormone changes during mirthful laughter. *Am J Med Sci*. 1989;298(6):390-6.

[107] Wooten, P. Humor: an antidote for stress. *Holist Nurs Pract*. 2996;10(2):49-56.

[108] Bennett MP, Lengacher C. Humor and laughter may influence health: III. Laughter and Health Outcomes. *Evid Based Complement Alternat Med*. 2008;5(1):37-40.

[109] Verghese J, Lipton R, Katz M, et al. Leisure Activities and the risk of dementia in the elderly. *N Engl J Med*. 2003;348(25):2508-2516.

[110] Bennett MP, Zeller JM, Rosenberg L, et al. The effect of mirthful laughter on stress and natural killer cell activity. *Altern Ther Health Med*. 2003;9(2):3845.

[111] Labott SM, Ahleman S, Wolever ME, et al. The physiological and psychological effects of the expression and inhibition of emotion. *Behav Med*. 1990;16(4):182-189.

[112] Chajes V, Thiebaut A, Rotival M, et al. Association between serum trans-monounsaturated fatty acids and breast cancer risk in the E3N-Epic Study. *Am J Epidemiol*. 2008;167(11):1312-1320.

[113] Goldberg IJ, Mosca L, Piano MR, Fisher EA. AHA Science Advisory: Wine and your heart: a science advisory for healthcare professionals from the Nutrition Committee, Council on Epidemiology and Prevention, and Council on Cardiovascular Nursing of the American Heart Association. *Circulation*. 2001; 103:472-5.

[114] Koppes LL, Dekker JM, Hendriks HF, Bouter LM, Heine RJ. Moderate alcohol consumption lowers the risk of type 2 diabetes: a meta-analysis of prospective observational studies. *Diabetes Care*. 2005; 28:719-25.

[115] Colotoni A, Emanuele MA, Kovacs EJ, et al. Hepatic estrogen receptors and alcohol intake. *Mol Cell Endocrinol*. 2007;193(1-2):101-4.

[116] Gong Z, Kristal AR, Schenk JM, et al. Alcohol consumption, finasteride, and prostate cancer risk: results from the Prostate Cancer Prevention Trial. *Cancer*. 2009;115(16):3661-9.

[117] Kraemer WJ, Ratamess NA. Hormonal responses and adaptations to resistance exercise and training. *Sports Med* 2005;35:339-361.

[118] Hackney AC. Effects of endurance exercise on the reproductive system of men: the "exercise-hypogonadal male condition." *J Endocrinol Invest* 2008;31:932-938.

[119] Penhollow T, Young M. Predictors of sexual satisfaction: the role of body image and fitness. *Electronic J Human Sexuality.* 2008. www.ejhs.org.

[120] Josefson D. Working the "graveyard" shift increases risk of colorectal cancer. *BMJ* 2003;326(7402):1286.

[121] Megdal SP, Kroenke CH, Laden F, et al. Night work and breast cancer risk: a systematic review and meta-analysis. *Eur J Cancer.* 2005;41(13)2023-32.

[122] Davis S, Mirick DK, Stevens RG. Night-shift work, light at night, and risk of breast cancer. *J Natl Cancer Inst* 2001;93:1557–62.

[123] Schernhammer ES, Laden F, Speizer FE, et al. Rotating night shifts and risk of breast cancer in women participating in the Nurses' Health Study. *J Natl Cancer Inst* 2001;93:1563–8.

[124] Moretti RM, Marelli MM, Maggi R, et al. Antiproliferative action of melatonin on human prostate cancer LNCaP cells. *Oncol Rep* 2000;7:347–51

[125] Straif K, Baan R, Grosse Y, Secretan B, et al. WHO International Agency for Research on Cancer Monograph Working Group. Carcinogenicity of shiftwork, painting, and fire-fighting. *The Lancet Oncology.* 2007;8:1065–1066.

[126]

[127] Schernhammer ES, Schulmeister K. Melatonin and cancer risk: does light at night compromise physiologic cancer protection by lowering serum melatonin levels? *Br J Cancer.* 2004;90(5):941-3.

[128] Najib T, et al. A prospective study of sleep duration and coronary heart disease in women. *Arch Intern Med* 2003;163:205-209.

[129] Gottlieb D, et al. Association of sleep time with diabetes mellitus and impaired glucose tolerance. *Arch Intern Med* 2005;165(8):863-7.

[130] Taheri S, Lin L, Austin D, et al. Short sleep duration is associated with reduced leptin, elevated ghrelin, and increased body mass index. *PLoS Med.* 2004;1(3):e62.

[131] Gangwisch JE, et al. Inadequate sleep as a risk factor for obesity: analyses of the NHANES I. *Sleep* 2005;29(10):1289-96.

[132] US EPA National Adipose Tissue Survey, 1982; EPA's Office of Prevention, Pesticides, and Toxic Substances, 1999.

[133] Stanley, JS, Ayling RE, Cramer PH, et al. Polychlorinated dibenzo-*p*-dioxin and dibenzofuran concentration levels in human adipose tissue samples from the continental United States collected from 1971 through 1987. *Chemosphere.* 1990;20(7-9):895-901.

[134] Body Burden, Environmental Working Group, 2005.

[135] US Environmental Protection Agency: 2000-2001 Pesticide Market Estimates: www.epa.gov/oppbead1/pestsales/01pestsales/usage2001.htm

[136] US EPA Toxic Release Inventory, Reporting Year 2008 National Analysis: Summary of Key Findings:

www.epa.gov/tri/tridata/tri08/national_analysis/pdr/TRI_key_findings_2008.pdf

[137] Beseler CL, Stallones L, Hoppin JA, et al. Depression and pesticide exposures among private pesticide applicators enrolled in the Agricultural Health Study. *Environ Health Perspect.* 2008;116(12): 1713-9

[138] Brown TP, Rumsby PC, Capleton AC, et al. Pesticides and Parkinson's disease — is there a link? *Environ Health Perspect.* 2006;114(2):156-64.

[139] Goldman LR. Managing pesticide chronic health risks: U.S. policies. *J Agromedicine.* 2007;12(1): 67-75.

[140] Hernandez AF, Casado I, Pena G, et al. Low level of exposure to pesticides leads to lung dysfunction in occupationally exposed subjects. *Inhal Toxicol.* 2008; 20(9): 839-49.

[141] Hoppin JA, Umbach DM, London SJ, et al. Pesticides and adult respiratory outcomes in the agricultural health study. *Ann N Y Acad Sci.* 2006;1076: 343-54.

[142] Bassil KL, Vakil C, Sanborn M, et al. Cancer health effects of pesticides: systematic review. *Can Fam Physician.* 2007;53(10): 1704-11.

[143] Alavanja MC, Ward MH, Reynolds P. Carcinogenicity of agricultural pesticides in adults and children. *J Agromedicine* 2007;12(1): 39-56.

[144] Andreotti G, Freeman LE, Hou L, et al. Agricultural pesticide use and pancreatic cancer risk in the Agricultural Health Study Cohort. *Int J Cancer* 2009;124(10):2495-500.

[145] Boobis A et al. Cumulative risk assessment of pesticide residues in food. *Toxicol Lett.* 2008; 180(2):137-50. Epub 2008 June 8

[146] Dodds EC, Lawson W. Synthetic oestrogenic agents without the phenanthrene nucleus. *Nature.* 1936;137:996.

[147] Bindhumol V, Chitra KC, Mathur PP. Bisphenol A induces reactive oxygen species generation in the liver of male rats. *Toxicology.* 2003;188(2-3):117-124.

[148] Nakagawa Y, Tayama S. Metabolism and cytotoxicity of bisphenol A and other bisphenols in isolated rat hepatocytes. *Arch Toxicol.* 2000;74(2):99-105.

[149] Moriyama K, Tagami T, Akamizu T, et al. Thyroid hormone action is disrupted by bisphenol A as an antagonist. *J Clin Endocrinol Metab.* 2002;87(11):5185-5190.

[150] Ropero AB, Alonso-Magdalena P, Garcia-Garcia E, Ripoll C, et al. Bisphenol-A disruption of the endocrine pancreas and blood glucose homeostasis. *Int J Androl.* 2008;31(2):194-200.

[151] Calafat AM, Ye X, Wong LY, et al. Exposure of the U.S. population to bisphenol A and 4-tertiary-octylphenol: 2003-2004. *Environ Health Perspect.* 2008;116(1):39-44.

[152] Carwile J, Luu H, Bassett L, et al. Polycarbonate bottle use and urinary bisphenol A concentrations. *Environ Health Perspectives*. 2009;117(9):1368-1372.

[153] Jensen TK, Toppari J, Keiding N, et al. Do environmental estrogens contribute to the decline in male reproductive health? *Clinic Chemistry*. 1995;41:1896-1901.

[154] Matsuda T, Abe H, Suda K. Relation between benign prostatic hyperplasia and obesity and estrogen [article in Japanese] *Rinsho Byori*. 2004;Apr;52(4):291-4.

[155] Wetherill YB, Fisher NL, Staubach A, et al. Xenoestrogen Action in Prostate Cancer: Pleiotropic Effects Dependent on Androgen Receptor Status. *Cancer Res*. 2005;65:54-65.

[156] Ilbarluzea J, Fernandez MF, Santa-Marina L, et al. Breast cancer risk and the combined effect of environmental estrogens. *Cancer Causes Control*. 2004;15(6):591-600.

[157] Louis GM, Weiner JM, Whitcomb BW, et al. Environmental PCB exposure and risk of endometriosis. *Hum Reprod*. 2005;20(1):279-85.

[158] Starek A. Estrogens and organochlorine xenoestrogens and breast cancer risk. *Int J Occup Med Environ Health*. 2003;16(2):113-24.

[159] Maffini MV. Endocrine disruptors and reproductive health: the case of bisphenol-A. *Mol Cell Endocrinol*. 2006;254-255:179-86.

[160] Diamanti-Kandarakis E, Bourguignon J, Giudice L, et al. Endocrine-disrupting chemicals: an endocrine society scientific statement. *Endocrine Reviews*. 2009;30(4):293-342.

[161] Environmental Working Group analysis of 97 canned foods, 2007.

[162] Janssen I, Ross R. Linking age-related changes in skeletal muscle mass and composition with metabolism and disease. *J Nutr Health Aging*. 2005 Nov-Dec;9(6):408-19.

[163] Van Pelt RE, Jones PP, Davy KP, et al. Regular exercise and the age-related decline in resting metabolic rate in women. *J Clin Endocrinol Metab*. 1997 Oct;82(10):3208-12.

[164] Van Pelt RE, Dinnerno FA, Seals DR, et al. Age-related decline in RMR in physically active men: relation to exercise volume and energy intake. *Am J Physiol Endocrinol Metab*. 2001 Sept;281(3):E633-9.

[165] Willcox DC, Willcox BJ, Todoriki H, et al. Caloric restriction and human longevity: What can we learn from the Okinawans? *Biogerontology*. 2006;7:173-77.

[166] Masoro E. Overview of caloric restriction and aging. *Mech Ageing Develop*. 2005;126(9):913-922.

[167] Fontana L, Klein S. Aging, Adiposity, and Calorie Restriction. *JAMA*. 2007;297:986-994.

[168] Calorie restriction. Shimizu T, Shirasawa T. Anti-aging effects by caloric restriction. [Article in Japanese] *Nippon Rinsho*. 2009:67(7):1366-71.

[169] Sacks FM, Bray GA, Carey VJ, et al. Comparison of weight-loss diets with different compositions of fat, protein, and carbohydrates. *N Engl J Med*. 2009;360(9):859-73.

[170] Thomas DE, Elliott EJ, Baur L. Low glycaemic index or low glycaemic load diets for overweight and obesity. *Cochrane Database Syst Rev*. 2007;18(3):CD005105.

[171] Saris W. Very-low-calorie diets and sustained weight loss. *Obesity Research*. 2001;Suppl 4:295S-301S.

[172] Wadden TA, West DS, Neierg RH, et al. One year weight losses in the Look AHEAD study: factors associated with success. *Obesity*. 2009;17(4):713-22.

[173] Crane FL. Discovery of ubiquinone (coenzyme Q) and an overview of function. *Mitochondrion*. 2007;Suppl:S2-7.

[174] Kalen A, Appelkvist EL, Dallner G. Age-related changes in the lipid compositions of rat and human tissues. *Lipids*. 1989;24(7):579-584.

[175] Ghirlanda G, et al. Evidence of plasma CoQ10-lowering effect by HMG-CoA reductase inhibitors: a double-blind, placebo-controlled study. *J Clin Pharmacol*.1993;33(3):226-9

[176] Quiles JL, Ochoa JJ, Battino M, et al. Life-long supplementation with a low dosage of coenzyme Q10 in the rat: effects on antioxidant status and DNA damage. *Biofactors*. 2005;25(1-4):73-86.

[177] Hodgson JM, Watts GF, Playford DA, et al. Coenzyme Q10 improves blood pressure and glycaemic control: a controlled trial in subjects with type 2 diabetes. *Eur J Clin Nutr*. 2002;56(11):1137-42.

[178] Dhanasekaran M, Ren J. The emerging role of coenzyme Q-10 in aging, neurodegeneration, cardiovascular disease, cancer and diabetes mellitus. *Curr Neurovasc Res*. 2005;2(5):447-59.

[179] Matthews RT, Yang L, Browne S, Baik M, Beal MF. Coenzyme Q10 administration increases brain mitochondrial concentrations and exerts neuroprotective effects. *Proc Natl Acad Sci USA*. 1998;95(15):8892-7.

[180] Rosenfeldt FL, Pepe S, Linnane A, et al. Coenzyme Q10 protects the aging heart against stress: studies in rats, human tissues, and patients. *Ann NY Acad Sci*. 2002;959:355-9.

[181] Wada H, Goto H, Hagiwara S, et al. Redox status of coenzyme Q10 is associated with chronological age. *J Am Geriatr Soc*. 2007;55(7):1141-2.

[182] Burr ML, Fehily AM, Gilbert JF et al. Effects of changes in fat, fish, and fibre intakes on death and myocardial reinfarction: diet and reinfarction trial (DART). *Lancet*. 1989;2(8666):75-61.

[183] Stone N. The Gruppo Italiano per lo Studio della Sopravvivenza nell'infarto miocardio (GISSI)-Prevenzione trial on fish oil and vitamin E supplementation in myocardial infarction survivors. *Current Cardiology Reports*. 2000;2(5):445-451.

[184] Saito Y, Yokoyama M, Origasa H, et al. Effects of EPA on coronary artery disease in hypercholesterolemic patients with multiple risk factors: subanalysis of primary prevention cases from the Japan EPA Lipid Intervention Study (JELIS). *Atherosclerosis*. 2008;2(1):135-140.

[185] Lavie CJ, Milani RV, Mehra MR, et al. Omega-3 polyunsaturated fatty acids and cardiovascular disease. *J Am Coll Cardiol* 2009; 54: 585-594.

[186] Colangelo LA, He K, Whooley MA, et al. Higher dietary intake of long-chain omega-3 polyunsaturated fatty acids is inversely associated with depressive symptoms in women. *Nutrition*. 2009;25(11):1011-9.

[187] Lin PY, Su KP. A meta-analytic review of double-blind, placebo-controlled trials of antidepressant efficacy of omega-3 fatty acids. *J Clin Psychiatry*. 2007;68(7):1056-61.

[188] Farzaneh-Far R, Lin J, Epel ES, et al. Association of marine omega-3 fatty acid levels with telomeric aging in patients with coronary heart disease. *JAMA*. 2010;303(3):250-7.

[189] Richards J, Valdes A, Gardner J, et al. Higher serum vitamin D concentrations are associated with longer leukocyte telomere length in women. *Am J of Clin Nutr*. 2007;86(5):1420-1425.

[190] D'Ambrosio D, Cippitelli M, Cocciolo MG, et al. Inhibition of IL-12 production by 1,25-dihydroxyvitamin D3. Involvement of NF-kappaB downregulation in transcriptional repression of the p40 gene. *J Clin Invest* 1998;101:252– 62.

[191] Puts MT, Visser M, Twisk J, et al. Endocrine and inflammatory markers as predictors of frailty. *Clin Endocrinol* 2005;63:403-11.

[192] Holick MF. Vitamin D deficiency: what a pain it is. *Mayo Clin Proc* 2003;78:1457-1459.

[193] Mouyis M, Ostor A, Crisp A, et al. Hypovitaminosis D among rheumatology outpatients in clinical practice. *Rheumatology*. 2008;47(9):1348-1351.

[194] Chowdhury TA, Boucher BJ, Hitman GA. Vitamin D and type 2 diabetes: is there a link? *Prim Care Diabetes*. 2009;3(2):115-6.

[195] Sood A, Arora R. Vitamin D deficiency and its correlations with increased cardiovascular incidences. *Am J Ther*. 2009 May 15 [Epub ahead of print].

[196] Zittermann A. Vitamin D and disease prevention with special reference to cardiovascular disease. *Prog Biophys Mol*. 2006;92(1):39-48.

[197] Zittermann A, Koerfer R. Vitamin D in the prevention and treatment of coronary heart disease. *Curr Opin Clin Nutr Metab Care*. 2008;11(6):752-7.

[198] Colston KW. Vitamin D and breast cancer risk. Best *Pract Res Clin Endocrinol Metab*. 2008;22(4):587-599.

[199] Blackmore KM, Lesosky M, Barnett H, et al. Vitamin D from dietary intake and sunlight exposure and the risk of hormone-receptor-defined breast cancer. *Am J Epidemiol*. 2008;168(8):915-24.

[200] Schwartz GG. Vitamin D and intervention trials in prostate cancer: from theory to therapy. *Ann Epidemiol*. 2009;19(2):96-102.

[201] Luong KV, Nguyen LT. The beneficial role of vitamin D and its analogs in cancer treatment and prevention. *Crit Rev Oncol Hematol*. 2009;May 14 [Epub ahead of print].

[202] Mizoue T, Kimura Y, Toyomura K, et al. Calcium, dairy foods, vitamin D, and colorectal cancer risk: the Fukuoka Colorectal Cancer study. *Cancer Epidemiol Biomarkers Prev*. 2008;17(10):2800-7.

[203] Marques F, Markus M, Morris B. Resveratrol: cellular actions of a potent natural chemical that confers a diversity of health benefits. *Int J Biochem Cell Biol*. 2009 [Epub ahead of print].

[204] Valenzano D, Terzibasi E, Genade T, et al. Resveratrol prolongs lifespan and retards the onset of age-related markers in a short-lived vertebrate. *Current Biology*. 2006;16:296-300.

[205] Baur JA, et al. Resveratrol improves health and survival of mice on a high-calorie diet. *Nature*. 2006:444(7117):337-42. Epub 2006 Nov 1.

[206] Zou JG, Wang ZR, Huang YZ, et al. Effect of red wine and wine polyphenol resveratrol on endothelial function in hypercholesterolemic rabbits. *Int J Mol Med*. 2003;11(3):317-20.

[207] Zbikowska HM, Olas B. Antioxidants with carcinostatic activity (resveratrol, vitamin E and selenium) in modulation of blood platelet adhesion. *J Physiol Pharmacol*. 2000;51(3):513-20.

[208] Pace-Asciak CR, Hahn S, Diamandis EP, et al. The red wine phenolics trans-resveratrol and quercetin block human platelet aggregation and eicosanoid synthesis: implications for protection against coronary heart disease. *Clin Chim Acta*. 1995;235(2):207-19.

[209] Sinha K, Chaudhary G, Gupta YK. Protective effect of resveratrol against oxidative stress in middle cerebral artery occlusion model of stroke in rats. *Life Sci*. 2002;71(6):655-65.

[210] Athar M, Back J, Kopelovich, et al. Multiple molecular targets of resveratrol: anti-carcinogenic mechanisms. *Arch Biochem Biophys* 2009:486(2):95-102.

[211] Boocoock D, Faust G, Patel K, et al. Phase I dose escalation pharmacokinetic study in healthy volunteers of resveratrol, a potential cancer chemopreventive agent. *Cancer Epidemiol Biomarkers Prev.* 2007;16(6):1246-52.

[212] Wong GY, Bradlow L, Sepkovic D, et al. Dose-ranging study of indole-3-carbinol for breast cancer prevention. *J Cell Biochem Suppl* 1997;28-29:111-6.

[213] Bell MC, Crowley-Norwick P, Bradlow HL, et al. Placebo-controlled trial of indole-3-carbinol in the treatment of CIN. *Gynecol Oncol* 2000;78:123-9.

[214] Jin L, Qi M, Chen DZ, et al. Indole-3-carbinol prevents cervical cancer in human papilloma virus type 16 (HPV16) transgenic mice. *Cancer Res.* 1999 Aug 15;59(16):3991-7.

[215] Degner SC, Papoutsis AJ, Selmin O, et al. Targeting of aryl hydrocarbon receptor-mediated activation of cyclooxygenase-2 expression by the indol-3-carbinol metabolite 3,3'-diindolymethane in breast cancer cells. *J Nutr.* 2009;139(1):26-32.

[216] Kristal AR, Lampe JW. Brassica vegetables and prostate cancer risk: a review of the epidemiological evidence. *Nutr Cancer* 2002;42(1):1-9.

[217] Muti P, Bradlow HL, Micheli A, et al. Estrogen metabolism and risk of breast cancer: a prospective study of the 2:16alpha-hydroxy-estrone ratio in premenopausal and postmenopausal women. *Epidemiology.* 2000 Nov;11(6):635-40.

[218] Bradlow HL, Telang NT, Sepkovic DW, Osborne MP. 2-hydroxyestrone: the 'good' estrogen. *J Endocrinol.* 1996 Sep;150 SupplS259-65.

[219] Dalessandri KM, Firestone GL, Fitch MD, Bradlow HL, Bjeldanes LF. Pilot study: effect of 3,3'-diindolylmethane supplements on urinary hormone metabolites in postmenopausal women with a history of early-stage breast cancer. *Nutr Cancer.* 2004;50(2):161-7.

[220] Fowke JH, Longcope C, Hebert JR. Brassica vegetable consumption shifts estrogen metabolism in healthy postmenopausal women. *Cancer Epidemiol Biomarkers Prev.* 2000 Aug;9(8):773-9

[221] Michnovicz JJ, Adlercreutz H, et al. Changes in levels of urinary estrogen metabolites after oral indol-3-carbinol treatment in humans. *J Natl Cancer Inst.* 1997;89(10):718-23.

[222] Report can be accessed through the FDA's website: http://www.fda.gov/Drugs/GuidanceComplianceRegulatoryInformation/PharmacyCompounding/ucm155725.htm

[223] Canonico M, Plu-Bureau G, Lowe GD, et al. Hormone replacement therapy and risk of venous thromboembolism in postmenopausal women: systematic review and meta-analysis. *BMJ*. 2008;336(7655):1227-31.

[224] Modena MG, Sismondi P, Mueck A, et al. New evidence regarding hormone replacement therapies is urgently required. Transdermal postmenopausal hormone therapy differs from oral hormone therapy in risks and benefits. *Maturitas*. 2005;52:1-10.

[225] Canonico M, Oger E, Plu-Bureau G, et al. Hormone therapy and venous thromboembolism among postmenopausal women. Impact of the route of estrogen administration and progestogens: the ESTHER study. *Circulation*. 2007;115:840-845.

[226] Glaser RL, Zava DT, Wurtzbacher D. Pilot study: absorption and efficacy of multiple hormones delivered in a single cream applied to the mucus membranes of the labia and vagina. *Gynecol Obstet Invest*. 2008;66(2):111-8.

[227] Bergkvist L, Hans-Olov A, Persson I, et al. The risk of breast cancer after estrogen and estrogen-progestin replacement. *N Engl J Med*. 1989;321:293-7.

[228] Million Women Study Collaborators. Breast cancer and hormone-replacement therapy in the Million Women Study. *Lancet*. 2003;362:419-27.

[229] Fournier A, Berrino F, Riboli E, et al. Breast cancer risk in relation to different types of hormone replacement therapy in the E3N-EPIC cohort. *Int J Cancer*. 2004;114:448-454.

[230] Rosenberg L, Magnusson C, Lindstrom E, et al. Menopausal hormone therapy and other breast cancer risk factors in relation to the risk of different histological subtypes of breast cancer: a case-control study. *Breast Ca Res*. 2006;8(1):1-13.

[231] Lyytinen H, Pukkala E, Ylikorkala O. Breast cancer risk in postmenopausal women using estrogen-only therapy. *Obstet Gynecol*. 2006;108(6):1354-1360.)

[232] Dew J, Wren B, Eden J. A cohort study of topical vaginal estrogen therapy in women previously treated for breast cancer. *Climacteric*. 2003;6:45-52.

[233] Glaser RL, Zava DT, Wurtzbacher D. Pilot study: absorption and efficacy of multiple hormones delivered in a single cream applied to the mucous membranes of the labia and vagina. *Gynecol Obstet Invest*. 2008;66(2):111-8.

[234] Labrie F, Luu-the V, Labrie C, et al. Endocrine and intracrine sources of androgens in women: inhibition of breast cancer and other roles of androgens and their precursor dehydroepiandrosterone. *Endocrine Reviews*. 2003;24(2):152-182.

[235] Glaser R, Wurtzbacher D, Dimitrakakis C. Efficacy of testosterone therapy deliverd by pellet implant. *Maturitas*. 2009;63:Suppl 1:S73-S74.

[236] Canonico M, Oger E, Plu-Bureau G, et al. Hormone therapy and venous thromboembolism among postmenopausal women: Impact of the route of estrogen administration and progestogens: the ESTHER Study. *Circulation.* 2007;115:840–5.

[237] Plu-Bureau G, Le MG, Thalabard JC, et al. Percutaneous progesterone use and risk of breast cancer: results from a French cohort study of premenopausal women with benign breast disease. *Cancer Detect Prev.* 1999;23(4):290-6.

[238] Fournier A, Berrino F, Clavel-Chapelon F. Unequal risks for breast cancer associated with different hormone therapies: results for the E3N cohort study. *Breast Cancer Res Treat.* 2008;107(1):103-111.

[239] Schumacher M, Coirini H, McEwen B. Regulation of high affinity GABA$_A$ receptors in the dorsal hippocampus by estradiol and progesterone. *Brain Res.* 1989;487:178–84.

[240] Leonetti HB, Wilson KJ, Anasti JN. Topical progesterone cream has an antiproliferative effect on estrogen-stimulated endometrium. *Fertil Steril.* 2003;79(1):221-2.

[241] Leonetti HB, Landes J, Steinberg D, et al. Transdermal progesterone cream as an alternative progestin in hormone therapy. *Altern Ther Health Med.* 2005;11(6):36-38.

[242] Leonetti HB, Longo S, Anasti JN. Transdermal progesterone cream for vasomotor symptoms and postmenopausal bone loss. *Obstet Gynecol.* 1999;94(2):225-8.

[243] Stephenson K, Price C, Kurdowska A, et al. Topical progesterone cream does not increase thrombotic and inflammatory factors in postmenopausal women. Presented at the 46th annual meeting of the American Society of Hematology, San Diego, Dec. 4-7, 2004. *Blood.* 2004;104(11 Pt 1):414b-415b.

[244] Andrade ES Jr, Clapauch R, Buksman S. Short term testosterone replacement therapy improves libido and body composition. *Arq Bras Endocrinol Metabol.* 2009;53(8):996-1004.

[245] Krapf JM, Simon JA. The role of testosterone in the management of hypoactive sexual disorder in postmenopausal women. *Maturitas.* 2009;63(3):213-9.

[246] Bolour S, Braunstein G. Testosterone therapy in women: a review. *Int J Impot Res.* 2005;17(5):399-408.

[247] Cardoza L, Gibb D, Tuck S, et al. The effects of subcutaneous hormone implants during the climacteric. *Maturitas.* 1984;5:177-184.

[248] Davis S, Goldstat R, Papalia M, et al. Effects of aromatase inhibition on sexual function and well-being in postmenopausal women treated with

testosterone: a randomized, placebo-controlled trial. *Menopause.* 2006;13(1):37-45.

[249] Pike C, Carroll J, Rosario E, et al. Protective actions of sex steroid hormones in Alzheimer's disease. *Frontiers in Neuroendocrinology.* 2009;30(2):239-258.

[250] Rosario E, Pike C. Androgen regulation of β-amyloid protein and the risk of Alzheimer's disease. *Brain Research Reviews.* 2008;57(2):444-453.

[251] Rako S. Testosterone deficiency: a key factor in the increased cardiovascular risk to women following hysterectomy or with natural aging? *J Womens Health.* 199;7(7):825-9.

[252] Worboys S, Kotsopoulos D, Teede H, et al. Evidence that parenteral testosterone therapy may improve endothelium-dependent and - independent vasodilation in postmenopausal women already receiving estrogen. *J Clin Endocrinol Metab.* 2001;86:158-161.

[253] Davis S, Walker S, Strauss B. Effects of estradiol with and without testosterone on body composition and relationships with lipids in postmenopausal women. *Menopause.* 2000;7(6):395-401.

[254] Dolan Looby SE, Collins M, Lee H, et al. Effects of long-term testosterone administration in HIV-infected women: a randomized, placebo-controlled trial. *AIDS.* 2009;23(8):951-959.

[255] Emmelot-Vonk M, Verhaar H, Nakhai Pour H, et al. Effect of testosterone supplementation on functional mobility, cognition, and other parameters in older men. *JAMA.* 2008;299(1):39-52.

[256] Miller KK, Biller BM, Hier J, et al. Androgens and bone density in women with hypopituitarism. *J Clin Endocrinol Metab.* 2002;87:2770-2776.

[257] Barlow DH, Abdalla HI, Roberts DR, et al. Long-term hormone implant therapy — hormonal and clinical effects. *Obstet Gynecol.* 1986;67:321.

[258] Davis S, McCloud P, Straus B, et al. Testosterone enhances estradiol's effects on postmenopausal bone density and sexuality. *Maturitas.* 1995;227-236.

[259] Cantrill JA, Dewis P, Large DM, et al. Which testosterone replacement therapy? *Clin Endocrinol (Oxf).* 1984; 21:97-107.

[260] Gooren L. New long-acting androgens. *World J Urol.* 2003;21:306-10

[261] DJ, Mackey MA, Howe C, et al. An analysis of testosterone implants for androgen replacement therapy. *Clin Endocrinol (Oxf)* 1997; 47: 311-6.

[262] Jockenhovel F, Vogel E, Kreutzer M, et al. Pharmacokinetics and pharmacodynamics of subcutaneous testosterone implants in hypogonadal men. *Clin Endocrinol (Oxf).* 1996;45:61-71.

[263] Vest S, Howard J. Clinical experiments with androgens. *JAMA.* 1939;113(21):1869-1872.

[264] Gambrell RD, Natrajan PK. Moderate dosage estrogen-androgen therapy improves continuation rates in postmenopausal women: impact of the WHI reports. *Climacteric*. 2006;9:224-233.

[265] Khastgir G, Studd J. Patient's outlook, experience, and satisfaction with hysterectomy, bilateral oophorectomy, and subsequent continuation of hormone replacement therapy. *Am J Obstet Gynecol*. 2000;183(6):1427-33.

[266] Handelsman DJ, Mackey MA, Howe C, et al. An analysis of testosterone implants for androgen replacement therapy. *Clin Endocrinol (Oxf)*. 1997;47:311-6.

[267] Jockenhovel F, Vogel E, Kreutzer M, et al. Pharmacokinetics and pharmacodynamics of subcutaneous testosterone implants in hypogonadal men. *Clin Endocrinol (Oxf)*. 1996;45;61-71.

[268] Davelaar EM, Gerretsen G, Relyveld J. [No increase in the incidence of breast carcinoma with subcutaneous administration of estradiol.] *Ned Tijdschr Geneeskd*. 1991;135(14):613-5.

[269] Dimitrakakis C, Jones R, Liu A, Bondy L. Breast cancer incidence in postmenopausal women using testosterone in addition to usual hormone therapy. *Menopause*. 2004;11(5):531-5.

[270] Natrajan P, Gambrell D. Estrogen replacement therapy in patients with early breast cancer. *Obstet Gynecol*. 2002;187:289-95.

[271] Natrajan P, Soumakis K, Gambrell D. Estrogen replacement therapy in women with previous breast cancer. *Obstet Gynecol*. 1999;181:288-295.

[272] Anderson C, Raju K, Forling M, Wheeler M. The effects of surgical menopause and parenteral hormone replacement therapy on bone density, menopausal symptoms, and hormone profiles. *Maturitas*. 1997;27(suppl 1):70.

[273] Barlow DH, Abdalla HI, Roberts DG, et al. Long-term hormone implant therapy – hormonal and clinical effects. *Obstet Gynecol*. 1986; 67:321.

[274] Davis S, McCloud P, Strauss B, et al. Testosterone enhances estradiol's effects on postmenopausal bone density and sexuality. *Maturitas*. 1995;227-236.

[275] Garnett T, Studd J, Watson N, et al. The effects of plasma estradiol levels on increases in vertebral and femoral bone density following therapy with estradiol and estradiol with testosterone implants. *Obstet Gynecol*. 1992;79:968-72.

[276] Garnett T, Studd J, Watson N, et al. A cross-sectional study of the effects of long-term percutaneous hormone replacement therapy on bone density. *Obstet Gynecol* 1991;78:1002-1007.

[277] Holland EF, Leather AT, Studd JW. The effect of 25-mg percutaneous estradiol implants on the bone mass of postmenopausal women. *Obstet Gynecol*. 1994;83:43-6.

[278] Khastgir G, Studd J, Holland N. Anabolic effect of estrogen replacement on bone in postmenopausal women with osteoporosis: histomorphometric evidence in a longitudinal study. *J Clin Endocrinol Metab*. 2001;86:289-295.

[279] Naessen T. Maintained bone density at advanced ages after long term treatment with low dose oestradiol implants. *Br J Obstet Gynecol*. 1993;100: 454-459.

[280] Notelovitz M, Johnston M, Smith S, et al. Metabolic and hormonal effects of 25-mg and 50-mg 17 beta-estradiol implants in surgically menopausal women. *Obstet Gynecol*. 1987;70:749.

[281] Notelovitz M. Androgen effects on bone and muscle. *Fertil Steril*. 2002;77(Suppl 4):S34-41.

[282] Pereda C, Hannon R, Naylor K, et al. The impact of subcutaneous oestradiol implants on biochemical markers of bone turnover and bone mineral density in postmenopausal women. *Br J Obstet Gynecol*. 2002;109:812-820.

[283] Savvas M, Studd J, Fogelman I, et al. Skeletal effects of oral oestrogen compared with subcutaneous oestrogen and testosterone in postmenopausal women. *BMJ*. 1988;297:331-333.

[284] Savvas M, Studd J, Norman S, et al. Increase in bone mass after one year of percutaneous oestradiol and testosterone implants in post-menopausal women who have previously received long-term oral estrogens. *Br J Obstet Gynecol*. 1992;99:757-760.

[285] Studd JW. The dose response of per-cutaneous oestradiol implants on the skeletons of postmenopausal women. *Br J Obstet Gynecol*. 1994;101:787-791.

[286] Vedi S, Purdie W, Ballard P, et al. Bone remodeling and structure in postmenopausal women treated with long-term, high-dose estrogen therapy. *Osteoporosis Int*. 1999;10:52-58.

[287] Magos A, Zilkha K, Studd K. Treatment of menstrual migraines by oestradiol implants. *J Neurol Neurosurg Psychiatry*. 1983;46:1044-46.

[288] Glaser R, Wurtzbacher D, Dimitrakakis C. Efficacy of testosterone therapy delivered by pellet implant. *Maturitas*. 2009;63(suppl 1):S73.

[289] Barlow DH, Abdalla HI, Roberts DG, et al. Long-term hormone implant therapy – hormonal and clinical effects. *Obstet Gynecol*. 1986; 67:321.

[290] Brincat M, Studd JW, O'Dowd T, et al. Subcutaneous hormone implants for the control of climacteric symptoms. *The Lancet*. 1984;16-18.

[291] Burger HG, Hailes J, Menelaus M, et al. The management of persistent menopausal symptoms with oestradiol-testosterone implants: clinical, lipid, and hormonal results. *Maturitas.* 1984;6:351-58.

[292] Cardozo L, Gibb D, Tuck S, et al. The effects of subcutaneous hormone implants during the climacteric. *Maturitas.* 1984;5:177-184.

[293] Montgomery J, Brincat M, Tapp A, et al. Effect of oestrogen and testosterone implants on psychological disorders in the climacteric. *The Lancet* 1987:297-299.

[294] Davis S, Walker K, Strauss B. Effects of estradiol with and without testosterone on body composition and relationships with lipids in postmenopausal women. *Menopause.* 2000;7(6):395-401.

[295] Lobo R, March C, Goebelsmann U, et al. Subdermal estradiol pellets following hysterectomy and oophorectomy. *Obstet Gynecol.* 1980;138:714-9.

[296] Worboys S, Kotsopoulos D, Teede H, et al. Evidence that parenteral testosterone therapy may improve endothelium-dependent and independent vasodilation in postmenopausal women already receiving estrogen. *J Clin Endocrinol Metab.* 2001;86:158-61.

[297] Maehle BO, Tretli S. Pre-morbid body-mass-index in breast cancer: reversed effect on survival in hormone receptor negative patients. *Breast Cancer Res Treat.* 1996;41(2):123-30.

[298] Morimoto LM, White E, Chen Z, et al. Obesity, body size, and risk of postmenopausal breast cancer: the Women's Health Initiative. *Cancer Causes Control.* 2002. 13(8):741-51.

[299] Gunter MJ, Hoover DR, Yu H, et al. Insulin, insulin-like growth factor-1, and risk of breast cancer in postmenopausal women. *J Natl Cancer Inst.* 2009;101(14):1030-1.

[300] Ness RB, Cauley JA. Antibiotics and breast cancer — what's the meaning of this? *JAMA.* 2004;291(7):880-881.

[301] Velicer CM, Heckbert SR, Lampe JW, et al. Antibiotic use in relation to the risk of breast cancer. *JAMA.* 2004;29(7):827-35.

[302] Mahmud K. Natural hormone therapy for menopause. *Gynecol Endorcrinol.* 2010;26(2):81-5.

[303] Rossouw JE, Anderson GL, Prentice RL, et al. Risks and benefits of estrogen plus progestin in healthy postmenopausal women. *JAMA.* 2002;288(3):321-333

[304] Beral V, Million Women Study Collaborators. Breast cancer and hormone-replacement therapy in the Million Women Study. *Lancet.* 2003;362(9382):419-27.

[305] Chen W, Manson J, Hankinson S, et al. Unopposed estrogen therapy and the risk of invasive breast cancer. *Arch Intern Med.* 2006;166:1027-1032.

[306] Davelaar EM, Gerretsen G, Relyveld J. [No increase in the incidence of breast carcinoma with subcutaneous administration of estradiol.] *Ned Tijdschr Geneeskd* 1991;135(14):613-5.

[307] Dimitrakakis C, Jones R, Liu A, Bondy L. Breast cancer incidence in postmenopausal women using testosterone in addition to usual hormone therapy. *Menopause* 2004;11(5):531-5.

[308] Natrajan P, Gambrell D. Estrogen replacement therapy in patients with early breast cancer. *Obstet Gynecol.* 2002;187:289-95.

[309] Somboonporn W, Davis S. Postmenopausal testosterone therapy and breast cancer risk. *Maturitas.* 2004;49:267-275.

[310] Bergkvist L, Hans-Olov A, Persson I, et al. The risk of breast cancer after estrogen and estrogen-progestin replacement. *N Engl J Med.* 1989;321:293-7.

[311] Million Women Study Collaborators. Breast cancer and hormone-replacement therapy in the Million Women Study. *Lancet.* 2003;362:419-27.

[312] Fournier A, Berrino F, Riboli E, et al. Breast cancer risk in relation to different types of hormone replacement therapy in the E3N-EPIC cohort. *Int J Cancer.* 2004;114:448-454.

[313] Rosenberg L, Magnusson C, Lindstrom E, et al. Menopausal hormone therapy and other breast cancer risk factors in relation to the risk of different histological subtypes of breast cancer: a case-control study. *Breast Ca Research.* 2006;8(1):1-13.

[314] Lyytinen H, Pukkala E, Ylikorkala O. Breast cancer risk in postmenopausal women using estrogen-only therapy. *Obstet Gynecol.* 2006;108(6):1354-1360.)

[315] Dew J, Wren B, Eden J. A cohort study of topical vaginal estrogen therapy in women previously treated for breast cancer. *Climacteric.* 2003;6:45-52.

[316] Keller PJ, Riedmann R, Fischer M, et al. Oestrogens, gonadotropins and prolactin after intra-vaginal administration of oestriol in post-menopausal women. *Maturitas.* 1981;3:47-53.

[317] Nahoul K, Dehennin L, Jondet M, et al. Profiles of plasma estrogens, progesterone, and their metabolites after oral or vaginal administration of estradiol or progesterone. *Maturitas.* 1993;16:185-202.

[318] Kuhl H. Pharmacology of estrogens and progestogens: influence of different routes of administration. *Climacteric.* 2005;8(suppl 1):3-63.

[319] Cowan LD, Gordis L, Tonascia J, et al. Breast cancer incidence in women with a history of progesterone deficiency. *Am J Epidemiol* 1981;114(2):209-17.

[320] Sturgeon S, Potischman N, Malone K, et al. Serum levels of sex hormones and breast cancer risk in premenopausal women: a case-control study. *Cancer Causes and Control.* 2004;15:45-53.

[321] Micheli A, Muti P, Secreto G, et al. Endogenous sex hormones and subsequent breast cancer in premenopausal women. *Int J Cancer.* 2004;112:312-318.

[322] Kaaks R, Berrino F, Key T, et al. Serum sex steroids in premenopausal women and breast cancer risk within the European Prospective Investigation into Cancer and Nutrition (EPIC). *J Natl Cancer Inst.* 2005;97:755-765.

[323] Plu-Bureau G, Le MG, Thalabard JC, et al. Percutaneous progesterone use and risk of breast cancer: results from a French cohort study of premenopausal women with benign breast disease. *Cancer Detect Prev.* 1993;23(4):290-6.

[324] Fournier A, Berrino F, Clavel-Chapelon F. Unequal risks for breast cancer associated with different hormone therapies: results for the E3N cohort study. *Breast Cancer Res Treat.* 2008;107(1):103-111.

[325] de Lignieres B, de Vathaire F, Fournier S, et al. Combined hormone replacement therapy and risk of breast cancer in a French cohort study of 3175 women. *Climacteric.* 2002;5:332-40.

[326] Somboonporn W, Davis S. Postmenopausal testosterone therapy and breast cancer risk. *Maturitas.* 2004;49:267-275.

[327] van Staa TP, Sprafka JM. Study of adverse outcomes in women using testosterone therapy. *Maturitas.* 2009;62(1):76-80.

[328] Hackenberg R, Schulz K. Androgen receptor mediated growth control of breast cancer and endometrial cancer modulated by antiandrogen and androgen-like steroids. *J Steroid Biochem Molec Biol.* 1996;56(1-6):113-117.

[329] Szelei J, Jimenez J, Soto A, et al. Androgen-induced inhibition of proliferation in human breast cancer MCF7 cells transfected with androgen receptor. *Endocrinology* 1997;138(4):1406-1412.

[330] Ortmann J, Prifti S, Bohlmann MK, et al. Testosterone and 5-alpha-dihydrotestosteorne inhibit in vitro growth of human breast cancer cell lines. *Gynecol Endocrinol.* 2002;16:113-120.

[331] Ando S, De Amicis F, Rago V, et al. Breast cancer: from estrogen to androgen receptor. *Molecular and Cellular Endocrinol.* 2002;193:121-128.

[332] Boccuzzi G, Brignardello E, DiMonaco M, et al. 5-En-androstne-3β, 17 β-diol inhibits the growth of MCF-7 breast cancer cells when oestrogen receptors are blocked by estradiol. *Br J Cancer.* 1994;70:1035-1039.

[333] Dimitrakakis C, Bondy C. Androgens and the breast. *Breast Cancer Res.* 2009;11(5):212.

[334] Szelei J, Jimenez J, Soto A, et al. Androgen-induced inhibition of proliferation in human breast cancer MCF7 cells transfected with androgen receptor. *Endocrinology* 1997;138(4):1406-1412.

[335] Kandouz M, Lombet A, Perrot J, et al. Proapoptotic effects of antiestrogens, progestins and androgen in breast cancer cells. *J Steroid Biochem Mol Biol.* 1999;69(1-6):463-71.

[336] Lapointe J, Fournier A, Richard V, et al. Androgens down-regulate bcl-2 protooncogene expression in ZR-75-1 human breast cancer cells. *Endocrinology.* 1999;140(1):416-421.

[337] Ando S, DeAmicis F, Rago V, et al. Breast cancer: from estrogen to androgen receptor. *Mol Cell Endocrinol.* 2002;193(1-2):121-8.

[338] Boccuzzi G, Brignardello E, Di Monaco M, et al. 5-en-androstene-3beta,17beta-diol inhibits the growth of MCF-7 breast cancer cells when oestrogen receptors are blocked by oestradiol. *Br J Cancer.* 1994;70:1035-1039.

[339] Zhou J, Ng S, Adesanya-Famuiya O, et al. Testosterone inhibits estrogen-induced mammary epithelial proliferation and suppresses estrogen receptor expression. *FASEB J.* 2000;14:1725–1730

[340] Poulin R, Baker D, Labrie F. Androgens inhibit basal and estrogen-induced cell proliferation in the ZR-75-1 human breast cancer cell line. *Breast Cancer Res Treat* 1988;12:213–225

[341] Langer M, Kubista E, Schemper M, et al. Androgen receptors, serum androgen levels and survival of breast cancer patients. *Arch Gynecol Obstet.* 1990;247:203-209.

[342] Bryan R, Mercer R, Bennett R, et al. Androgen receptors in breast cancer. *Cancer.* 2006;54(11):2436-2440.

[343] Tormey DC, Lippman ME, Edwards BK, et al. Evaluation of tamoxifen doses with and without fluoxymesterone in advanced breast cancer. *Ann Intern Med.* 2003;98:139–144

[344] Ingle JN, Twito DI, Schaid DJ, et al. Combination hormonal therapy with tamoxifen plus fluoxymesterone *vs.* tamoxifen alone in postmenopausal women with metastatic breast cancer. A phase II study. *Cancer.* 1991;67:886–891

[345] Birrell S, Butler L, Harris J, et al. Disruption of androgen receptor signaling by synthetic progestins may increase risk of developing breast cancer. *FASEB Journal.* 2007;21:2285-2293.

[346] Zhou J, Ng S, Adesanya-Famuiya A, et al. Testosterone inhibits estrogen-induced mammary epithelial proliferation and suppresses estrogen receptor expression. *FASEB Journal.* 2000;14:1725-1730.

[347] Hoffling M, Hirschberg A, Skoog L, et al. Testosterone inhibits estrogen/progestogen-induced breast cell proliferation in postmenopausal women. *Menopause.* 2007;14(2):1-8.

[348] Dimitrakakis C, Zhou J, Wang J, et al. A physiologic role for testosterone in limiting estrogenic stimulation of the breast. *Menopause.* 2003;10(4):292-298.

[349] Natrajan P, Gambrell D. Estrogen replacement therapy in patients with early breast cancer. *Am J Obstet Gynecol.* 2002;187:289-95.

[350] Cottet V, Touvier M, Fournier A, et al. Postmenopausal breast cancer risk and dietary patterns in the E3N-EPIC prospective cohort study. *Am J Epidemiol.* 2009;170(10):1257-67.

[351] Smith–Warner SA, Spiegelman D, Yaun SS, et al. Alcohol and breast cancer in women: a pooled analysis of cohort studies. *JAMA* 1998; 279:535-40.

[352] Cummings SR, Tice JA, Bauer S, et al. Prevention of breast cancer in postmenopausal women: approaches to estimating and reducing risk. *J Natl Cancer Inst.* 2009;101(6):384-98.

[353] McTiernan A, Kooperberg C, White E, et al. Recreational physical activity and the risk of breast cancer in postmenopausal women: The Women's Health Initiative Cohort Study. *JAMA.* 2003; 290(10):1331–1336.

[354] Collaborative Group on Hormonal Factors in Breast Cancer. Breast cancer and breastfeeding: collaborative reanalysis of individual data from 47 epidemiological studies in 30 countries, including 50302 women with breast cancer and 96973 women without the disease. *Lancet.* 2002;360(9328):187-195.

[355] Yang L, Jacobsen KH. A systematic review of the association between breastfeeding and breast cancer. *J Womens Health (Larchmt).* 2008;17(10):1635-1645.

[356] Maehle BO, Tretli S. Pre-morbid body-mass-index in breast cancer: reversed effect on survival in hormone receptor negative patients. *Breast Cancer Res Treat.* 1996;41(2):123-30.

[357] Morimoto LM, White E, Chen Z, et al. Obesity, body size, and risk of postmenopausal breast cancer: the Women's Health Initiative. *Cancer Causes Control.* 2002. 13(8):741-51.

[358] Gunter MJ, Hoover DR, Yu H, et al. Insulin, insulin-like growth factor-1, and risk of breast cancer in postmenopausal women. *J Natl Cancer Inst.* 2009;101(14):1030-1.

[359] Terry P, Rohan T. Cigarette smoking and the risk of breast cancer in women: a review of the literature. *Cancer Epidemiol Biomarkers Prev.* 2002;11:953-971.

[360] Antoni MH, Lutgendorf SK, Cole SW, et al. The influence of bio-behavioural factors on tumour biology: Pathways and mechanisms. *Nat Rev Cancer.* 2006; 6(3):240–248.

[361] John EM, Schwartz GG, Dreon DM, et al. Vitamin D and breast cancer risk: the NHANES I epidemiologic follow-up study, 1971-1975 to 1992. National Health and Nutrition Examination Survey. *Cancer Epidemiol Biomarkers Prev.* 1999;8(5):399-406.

[362] Lappe JM, Travers-Gustafson D, Davies KM, et al. Vitamin D and calcium supplementation reduces cancer risk: results of a randomized trial. *Am J Clin Nutr.* 2007;85(6):1586-91.

[363] Gray J, Evans N, Taylor B, et al. State of the evidence: the connection between breast cancer and the environment. *Int J Occup Environ Health.* 2009;15(1):43-78.

[364] Wong GY, Bradlow L, Sepkovic D, et al. Dose-ranging study of indole-3-carbinol for breast cancer prevention. *J Cell Biochem Suppl* 1997;28-29:111-6.

[365] Sun CL, Yuan JM, Koh WP, et al. Green tea, black tea and breast cancer risk: a meta-analysis of epidemiological studies. *Carcinogenesis.* 2006;27(7):1310-5.

[366] Seely D, Mills EJ, Verma S, et al. The effects of green tea consumption on incidence of breast cancer and recurrence of breast cancer: s systematic review and meta-analysis. *Integr Cancer Ther.* 2005;4(2)144-55.

[367] Cos S, Fernandez F, Sanchez-Barcelo EJ. Melatonin inhibits DNA synthesis in MCF-7 human breast cancer cells in vitro. *Life Sci.* 1996;58(26):2447-53.

[368] Ram PT, Yuan L, Dai J. Differential responsiveness of MCF-7 human breast cancer cell line stocks to the pineal hormone, melatonin. *J Pineal Res.* 2000;28(4):210-8.

[369] Subramanian A, Kothari L. Suppressive effect by melatonin on different phases of 9,10-dimethyl-1,2-benzanthracene (DMBA)-induced rat mammary gland carcinogenesis. *Anticancer Drugs.* 1991;2(3):297-303.

[370] Schernhammer ES, Hankinson SE. Urinary melatonin levels and postmenopausal breast cancer risk in the Nurses' Health Study cohort. *Cancer Epidemiol Biomarkers Prev.* 2009;18(1):74-9.

[371] Goodstine Sh, Zheng T, Holford T, et al. Dietary ($\Omega$-3)/($\Omega$-6) fatty acid ratio: possible relationship to premenopausal but not postmenopausal breast cancer risk in US women. *J. Nutr.* 2003;133:1409-1414.

[372] KIim J, Lim SY, Shin A, et al. Fatty fish and fish omega-3 fatty acid intakes decrease the breast cancer risk: a case-control study. *BMC Cancer.* 2009;9:216.

[373] Tamimi RM, Colditz GA, Hankinson SE. Circulating carotenoids, mammographic density, and subsequent risk of breast cancer. *Cancer Res.* 2009;69(24):9323-9329.

[374] Shen J, Gammon MD, Terry MB, et al. Telomere length, oxidative damage, antioxidants, and breast cancer risk. *Int J Cancer.* 2009;124(7):1637-1643.

[375] American Institute for Cancer Research & World Cancer Research Fund, 2007

[376] Giovannucci E. A review of epidemiologic studies of tomatoes, lycopene, and prostate cancer. *Exp Biol Med.* 2002;227:852-859.

[377] Vogt TM, Mayne ST, Graubard BI, et al. Serum lycopene, other serum carotenoids, and risk of prostate cancer in US Blacks and Whites. *Am J Epidemiol.* 2002;155:1023-1032.

[378] Snowdon D, Phillips R, Choi W. Diet, obesity, and risk of fatal prostate cancer. *Am J Epidemiol.* 1984;120(2):244-250.

[379] Amling CL. Relationship between obesity and prostate cancer. *Curr Opin Urol.* 2005;15(3):167-71.

[380] Ma RW, Chapman K. A systemic review of the effect of diet in prostate cancer prevention and treatment. *J Hum Nutr Diet* 2009;22:187-199.

[381] Heinonen OP, Albanes D, Virtamo J, et al. Prostate cancer and supplementation with alpha-tocopherol and beta-carotene: incidence and mortality in a controlled trial. *J Natl Cancer Inst* 1998;90(6):440-6.

[382] Crispen PL, Uzzo RG, Golovine K, et al. Vitamin E succinate inhibits NF-kappaB and prevents the development of a metastatic phenotype in prostate cancer cells: implications for chemoprevention. *Prostate.* 2007;67(6):582-90.

[383] Lippman SM, Klein EA, Goodman PJ, et al. Effect of selenium and vitamin E on risk of prostate cancer and other cancers: the selenium and vitamin E cancer prevention trial (SELECT). *JAMA.* 2009;30(1):39-51.

[384] Etminan M, FitzGerald M, Gleave M, et al. Intake of selenium in the prevention of prostate cancer: a systematic review and meta-analysis. *Cancer Causes Control.* 2005;16(9):1125-31.

[385] Li H, Stampfer MJ, Giovannucci EL, et al. A prospective study of plasma selenium levels and prostate cancer risk. *J Natl Cancer Inst.* 2004;96:696-703.

[386] Duffield-Lillico AJ, Dalkin BL, Reid ME, et al. Selenium supplementation, baseline plasma selenium status and incidence of prostate cancer: an analysis of the complete treatment period of the Nutritional Prevention of Cancer Trial. *BJU Int.* 2003;91:608-612.

[387] Combs GF, Jr. Status of selenium in prostate cancer prevention. *Br J Cancer.* 2004;91:195-199.

[388] Brooks JD, Metter EJ, Chan DW, et al. Plasma selenium level before diagnosis and the risk of prostate cancer development. *J Urol.* 2001;166:2034-2038.

[389] Yoshizawa K, Willett WC, Morris SJ, et al. Study of prediagnostic selenium level in toenails and the risk of advanced prostate cancer. *J Natl Cancer Inst.* 1998;90:1219-1224.

[390] Chen TC, Holick MF. Vitamin D and prostate cancer prevention and treatment. *Trends Endocrinol Metab.* 2003;14(9):423-30.

[391] Ahonen MH, Tenkanen L, Teppo L, et al. Prostate cancer risk and prediagnostic serum 25-hydroxyvitamin D levels. *Cancer Causes Control.* 2000;11(9):847-52.

[392] Giovannucci E, Liu Y, Rimm EB, Hollis BW, et al. Prospective study of predictors of vitamin D status and cancer incidence and mortality in men. *J Natl Cancer Inst.* 2006;98(7):451-9.

[393] Roddam AW, Allen NE, Appleby P, et al. Endogenous sex hormones and prostate cancer: a collaborative analysis of 18 prospective studies. *J Natl Cancer Inst.* 2008;100:170-83.

[394] Morgentaler A, Bruning CO, DeWolf WC. Occult prostate cancer in men with low serum testosterone levels. *JAMA.* 1996;276:1904-6.

[395] Morgentaler A, Rhoden EL. Prevalence of prostate cancer among hypogonadal men with PSA of 4.0ng/mL or less. *Urology.* 2006;68:1263-67.

[396] Imamoto T, Suzuki H, Fukasawa S, et al. Pretreatment serum testosterone level as a predictive factor of pathological stage in localized prostate cancer patients treated with radical prostatectomy. *Eur Urol.* 2005;47:308-12.

[397] Schatzl G, Madersbacher S, Thurridl T, et al. High-grade prostate cancer is associated with low serum testosterone levels. *Prostate.* 2001;47:52-8. & Yano M, Imamoto T, Suzuki H, et al. The clinical potential of pretreatment serum testosterone level to improve the efficiency of prostate cancer screening. *Eur Urol.* 2007;51:375-80.

[398] Massengill JC, Sun L, Moul JW, et al. Pretreatment total testosterone level predicts pathological stage in patients with localized prostate cancer treated with radical prostatectomy. *J Urol.* 2003;169:1670-5.

[399] Isom-Batz G, Bianco Jr FJ, KattanMW, et al. Testosterone as a predictor of pathological stage in clinically localized prostate cancer. *J Urol.* 2005;173:1935-7

[400] Yamamoto S, Yonese J, Kawakami S, et al. Preoperative serum testosterone level as an independent predictor of treatment failure following radical prostatectomy. *Eur Urol* 2007;52:696-701.

[401] Marks LS, Mazer NA, Mostaghel E, et al. Effect of testosterone replacement therapy on prostate tissue in men with late-onset hypogonadism: a randomized controlled trial. *JAMA* 2006;296:2351-61.

[402] Hernandez B, Park S, Wilkens L, et al. Relationship of body mass, height, and weight gain to prostate cancer risk in the multiethnic cohort. *Cancer Epidemiol Biomarkers Prev.* 2009;18(9):2413-21.

[403] Brunoni AR, Lopes M, Fregni F. A systematic review and meta-analysis of clinical studies on major depression and BDNF levels: implications for the

role of neuroplasticity in depression. *Int J Neuropsychopharmacol.* 2008;11(8):1169-80.

[404] Cotman CW, Berchtold NC. Exercise: a behavioral intervention to enhance brain health and plasticity. *Trends Neurosci.* 2002;25(6):295-301.

[405] Laske C, Banschbach S, Stransky, et al. Exercise-induced normalization of decreased BDNF serum concentration in elderly women with remitted major depression. *Int J Neuropsychopharmacol.* 2010;13:1-8. [Epub ahead of print]

[406] Tyler WJ, Alonso M, Bramham CR, et al. From acquisition to consolidation: on the role of brain-derived neurotrophic factor signaling in hippocampal-dependent learning. *Learn Mem.* 2002;9(5):224-37.

[407] Oliff HS, Berchtold NC, Isackson P, et al. Exercise-induced regulation of brain-derived neurotrophic factor (BDNF) transcripts in the rat hippocampus. *Brain Res Mol Brain Res.* 1998;61(1-2):147-53.

[408] Logan AC. Omega-3 and BDNF regulation: eicosapentaenoic acid may play a key role in limitation of CNS injury. *J Neurotrauma.* 2008;25(12):1499.

[409] Garcion E, Wion-Barbot N, Montero-Menei C, et al. New clues about vitamin D functions in the nervous system. *Trends Endocrin Metab.* 2002;13(2):100-105.

[410] Scharfman H, MacLusky N. Estrogen and brain-derived neurotrophic factor (BDNF) in hippocampus: complexity of steroid hormone-growth factor interactions in the adult CNS. *Front Neuroendocrinol.* 2006;27(4):415-35.

[411] Gold SM, Voskuhl RR. Testosterone replacement therapy for the treatment of neurological and neuropsychiatric disorders. *Curr Opin Investig Drugs.* 2006;7(7):625-30.

[412] Bialek M, Zaremba P, Borowicz KK, et al. Neuroprotective role of testosterone in the nervous system. *Pol J Pharmacol.* 2004;56(6):509-18.

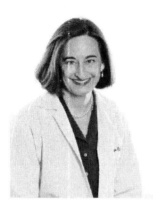

Kathryn Retzler, ND is a naturopathic physician and an authority on natural medicine and hormone balance. She draws on both conventional and alternative therapies and believes that people benefit most from a blend of all available treatments, focused on individual needs. Dr. Retzler has served as a consultant and lecturer to other physicians and pharmacists about hormone testing, bioidentical hormone replacement, and neurotransmitter optimization. She understands the role balanced hormones and neurotransmitters play in all areas of health and recommends natural therapies, lifestyle changes and bioidentical hormones to address the underlying causes of hormone imbalance and restore health and vitality.

Dr. Retzler lives in Portland, Oregon with her husband, Daniel, and two dogs, Libby and Baraka.